For my mother,

whose love made me who I am

"Nothing in life is to be feared. It is only to be understood."
Marie Curie

"Each patient carries his own doctor inside him. We are at our best when we give that doctor who resides in us a chance to work."
Albert Schweitzer

Copyright © 2019 Tamara Gurin. All Rights Reserved.

Table of Contents

Foreword 6
Chapter 1. How It Started 11
   Dr. B 11
   Aunt Gina 13
   Vacation 15
   Downward Spiral 16
   Before You Move On 19
Chapter 2. The Maze 21
   Chiropractor Sandy 21
   Acupressure. The Kathleen 23
   Stuck 25
   Nerves Are Very Logical 30
   Second Opinion 32
   Against the Brick Wall 34
   Physical Therapy 36
   Acupuncture 38
   Lifeline 41
Chapter 3. Rock Bottom 46
   The Wall Is Getting Taller and Denser 46
   Downward Spiral Continues 48
   Hope Crashed 49
   Diagnosis 54

Chapter 4. Awakening ... 59
  Fateful Day ... 59
  Mindbody and TMS ... 60
  Forums ... 64
  Nothing Is Wrong With My Body – But How Do I Know? 68
  It Is All in My Head ... 70
  Thank you, Dr. L ... 71
  Thinking Psychologically ... 74
  Throwing Away Crutches ... 77
  Forum of Hope ... 78
  TMS Practitioners ... 80
Chapter 5. Healing and Recovery ... 84
  The Toolbox ... 84
  Cure vs. Healing ... 85
  Insomnia ... 89
  Mindfulness ... 91
  Meditation ... 93
  Sitting Meditation ... 96
  Running Meditation ... 98
  Yoga ... 102
  Qi Gong ... 104
  Overcoming Fear ... 105
  Faith ... 107
  Feeling Stuck ... 112
  Non-Linear Recovery and Extinction Bursts ... 115

Plateau 118

Frozen Emotions 119

Dr. Render, Osteopath 124

Dr. Farias 128

Acupressure and Qi 132

Support Team 134

Journaling 137

Encouragement, Reassurance, and Celebration 138

Phobias 140

Chapter 6. Summary 142

Timeline 142

What I Learned 145

Is a Complete Recovery Possible? 146

Official Diagnosis 148

Square Peg in the Round Hole 151

Confident Doctors and Over-Confident Doctors 154

Faith, Patience, Courage 155

Glossary 158

Bibliography 160

Foreword

I am not a writer. I never intended to write books until I found myself a witness to a stunning recovery from a very crippling and, per official medicine, incurable illness – my own recovery. My experience defied the official statistics and was so convincing that I decided that it could help others with neurological conditions to read my story.

If somebody had told me before the year 2016 that such a path to recovery was possible, I would have responded with great skepticism. As I look back at my journey, some of the things that happened to me seem like they came from a fictional story – but I know they were true; my medical records, notes, and letters are evidence to that.

I am not a scientist. After I became sick, my understanding of neuroscience and psychology grew substantially, from almost zero to a fair amount. However, I still do not possess knowledge to even remotely qualify as a researcher. None of the statements made in this book should be viewed as formal research. It is just a set of observations, based mostly on a single subject – myself. Yet, as I was looking for the ways to heal, I was in contact with many people who had traveled a similar path out of their illness - and succeeded.

I am not a healthcare professional. I am not giving anyone any medical advice, let alone a recommendation, on how or even whether to seek a non-orthodox way to cure their illness. Even more so, this book is not advice to those who are suffering from a rapidly progressing terminal condition like cancer. However, I would like to document and publish evidence of how I healed myself from a supposedly incurable illness and of all the help I used along the way because it may help some of those in a desperate need for help.

I am also hoping that this book will be read by a doctor (or even more than a few doctors!) who are interested in a patient's view on the healing process. It is a long shot, but I am still hoping that maybe some doctors will be able to revisit the ways they diagnose and treat neurological conditions.

As I navigated through the maze of our healthcare system, sometimes with hope, sometimes with relief, but more frequently with fear and bewilderment, I promised myself that if recovered, I would write a guidebook for those who are still wandering in the maze. As I worked on this book, I came to realization that a step-by-step guidebook on how to recover from a neurological disease should not be written, primarily because each person is unique and should follow their own path.

In the end, the book turned out to be not a set of specific instructions that should be followed, but rather a story of my own recovery that may be useful to others, as it was a path of trial and error, but also a path of determination and faith.

All my life experiences, my education, and my profession prepared me not to believe in miracles. I have always relied on facts, proofs, and argumentation leading to logical conclusions. However, I am realizing that, unlike my professional field of software engineering, where most of the mysteries can be tracked down and explained by provable facts, the field of clinical medicine operates in a significantly more complex world with many more variables and with the subjects of study invariably more complex than computers. Therefore, there is much more room for unexplained and unexplainable, and the stakes are so much higher. As a result, practitioners must be by far more risk-averse than software engineers. However, I came out of my illness with the feeling that in addition to being complex due to its nature, our healthcare system is unreasonably overcomplicated, which makes it less efficient and certainly more resource intensive, to the detriment of all of us, who are all but guaranteed to have to deal with the healthcare system sooner or later in our lives.

I also learned a great deal about faith, which I used to discard as something immaterial and immeasurable, therefore something that should not even be considered when dealing with facts. My own experience made me revisit my prior convictions and made me learn about the power of faith. It is the newfound understanding of the power of faith in myself that changed my life.

So, to those who may have picked up this book in search for precise how-to instructions on recovery from neurological conditions, my advice would be not to look for instructions and not to follow my path exactly step by step. Chart your own journey, be brave, and try any opportunity that comes your way. Don't be afraid to keep what works and discard what does not.

I would like to express my deepest gratitude to many people who helped me on my way:

To Dr. John E. Sarno, whose courage to go against the flow and not shy away from a controversy, whose determination to ask questions and seek answers changed so many lives, including my own.

To Alan Gordon, Director of Pain Psychology Center in LA, who continues Dr. Sarno's work through the TMS Wiki and TMS Forum, for his outstanding service to the community.

To the people on the TMS Forum (www.tmswiki.org/forum), whose knowledge, kindness, and wisdom guided me to my recovery: plum, balto, Ellen, JanAtheCPA, Eric Watson, and many others. Some of your real names I may never know, but I will never forget your advice and your compassion so generously given to me when I desperately needed it. Without you, I would never have made the recovery and would never find the wisdom and knowledge that will stay with me for the rest of my life. I will always try to give back.

To Kathleen Davis, for her wisdom, kindness, and generosity to her students, clients, and friends.

To Steve Myers, my dear friend, partner, running coach, and inspiration, for quietly stepping in to help me when I was nearly disabled.

To Amber Murphy, my cheerleader and supporter, who helped me lose fear and find faith in myself.

To Dr. Roger Gietzen, for helping me clear the fog and confusion and for encouraging me to write about my experience.

To Dr. Rebecca Render, for her determination to try, explore, and never give up, her love for her patients and her radiant smile that greets me each time I come to see her.

To my friends from the acupressure community for your support and encouragement: Panda, Aline, Janice, Min.

To my son, Ilya, my strict and demanding editor and my backpacking partner, for always challenging me to overcome my fears.

To Deborah Smith Lawrence, for her wisdom and infinite kindness.

To Google search engine, for helping so many to find information otherwise hidden from us. Knowledge is power.

My special heartfelt thanks to my informal editorial board: Roger Geitzen, M.D. and Panda Hershey, Ph.D., for your invaluable and generous contribution to this book. Your feedback, thoughts and comments made it so much better!

In consideration for privacy, some of the names in the book have been modified. The name of my healthcare provider The Clinic in the book is not a real name.

Chapter 1. How It Started

Dr. B

September 24, 2015 was supposed to be just a usual busy Thursday, but something unusual happened that day. I woke up with a strange feeling in my left arm. It was swollen from the wrist to the elbow, and my middle finger curled in and was stuck in that position. The arm was painful from swelling. I had never experienced anything like that before.

I scheduled an appointment with my doctor at The Clinic, Dr. B, and went to see her the following week.

I like The Clinic. I like its sprawling campus in my town. The buildings are clean, modern-looking, and well-decorated. The courtyard has bamboo plants and a rock garden and waiting rooms are cozy and comfortable.

I love The Clinic's computer system. My prescription appears at the pharmacy as soon as the doctor finishes typing it in, I can see my test results on the web site a few hours after I leave the lab, I can access to the doctors via email. I like The Clinic's staff. Receptionists are efficient, friendly and full of sympathy for sick people. They go the extra mile for you to meet your needs. They usually say: "we don't want you to be unhappy" – and get things done for you: expedite your appointments or get you back in line if you stepped out and missed your call to the doctor.

Dr. B. was a pleasant woman in her late 30-s; we got along quite well. She has a pleasant smile and subtle sense of humor. When choosing her as my primary physician, I sifted through the profiles of the doctors on The Clinic web site and selected the one that shared my philosophy. This is what she wrote: "While I can recommend life changes, tests, and medication, most of the work and rewards are up to you." I, too, believe that my health belongs to me, not my doctors. I do not believe in magic pills, and I practice yoga, exercise, and eat healthy – so even in my 60s I can hike 25 miles a day, swim a mile or two, and beat some young punks to the mountain peaks.

For years, I did not bother Dr. B much with my health problems, other than a sudden onset of vertigo a few years back, which she fixed by looking things up on her computer and then artfully performing the Epley maneuver on me.

When we first met, I did complain about my decades-old insomnia, but other than prescribing me a sleep medication that was as useless as the other sleep medications prescribed to me before, she could not come up with any alternatives, and we agreed that I just had to live with insomnia.

The bottom line, I got along with The Clinic and Dr. B just fine.

Until I got sick.

As I entered her office, Dr. B was all smiles, as usual. She did not think much of my illness. Ever confident, she determined that I had a carpal tunnel syndrome and asked if I had some unusual physical activity in the preceding weeks. I was relieved that it was something so basic but expressed doubts about the diagnosis. In my opinion, I had not had any repetitive movements that could overwork my wrist. Maybe, scraping paint off my deck a couple weeks prior to this episode, but nothing immediately preceding the swelling and pain. Dr. B was undeterred by my timid arguments. With her usual pleasant smile, she prescribed me a brace, recommended I go easy on my wrist, and assured me that I would soon forget the pain, for as long as I followed her instructions. And so I dutifully did, for a few weeks. The pain did slow down, but the fingers remained as curled as they were on day one.

Five weeks after the initial incident, I left for vacation in Spain, equipped with my brace and determination to give my wrist all the rest it needed. In my two weeks in Spain filled with hiking and sightseeing, I lifted nothing heavier than a coffee cup with my hand – OK, I also lifted my day pack; I did almost no cooking and absolutely no typing or paint scraping. Nevertheless, my fingers were still painful and curled. They didn't seem to respond to the prescribed rest.

I became increasingly worried. My worries were amplified by the memories of my grandaunt.

Aunt Gina

Aunt Gina was my mother's aunt. I first met her when I was 8. When I was 13 and she was in her 70s, we moved to the town where she lived and where she retired from a long career as a dentist. Never married, she invested her life in her nieces, nephews, and their children. With bright blue eyes and gray hair in a bun, she was intelligent, energetic, and invariably optimistic, despite a very hard life and many illnesses, from severe asthma and diabetes to the mysterious strain of Parkinson's, which she was diagnosed with in her late 60s.

Her Parkinson's was quite atypical: She did not have any tremors or loss of balance, or even a minor cognitive decline. Her back was straight, speech clear and confident, and her head was in perfect order. She could go on for hours telling stories of her life and reciting numerous poems she had learned in grade school. As far as Parkinson's goes, she had just two symptoms: Her left hand was squeezed in a fist and her entire arm was extremely painful. Her illness progressed rather rapidly, and soon her left leg became stiff and rigid and she started limping. Her hand meanwhile, was getting tighter and tighter, and it took her a tremendous effort to pull her fingers apart. As soon as her fingers were not held open by force, they would immediately collapse into a fist. Eventually, her left elbow was bent and pushed into her ribs by the same mysterious force, and pain became a constant presence, especially at night.

Eventually her left side was mostly paralyzed and night pain became unbearable. Painkillers did not help much. She was a tough, strong woman who grew up in poverty and lived through wars and famines. But even she could not cope with this merciless enemy that, having paralyzed her left side, started making inroads on her right side, gradually taking control of her right hand, arm, and leg.

By the time she was 85, she was begging for death to come. Unfortunately, her heart continued to work flawlessly, and her mind was still completely lucid. She died in her 90s.

Since we lived nearby, I helped to take care of her. The sight of her gradually becoming more and more incapacitated and unable to take care of herself was a constant presence in my life until I was in my mid-30s. I remember the sense of helplessness when I sat by her bedside. All we could do was listen to her and listening while not being able to help was torturous.

In September of 2015, when I first realized that my middle finger curled in and would not open, one of the first thoughts that came to my mind was that maybe I, too, had

Parkinson's. Fear of incurable and devastating illness scared me, but I brushed it off. So, I was very relieved to learn from Dr. B about the diagnosis. Carpal tunnel was a much, much better outcome than the slow, unstoppable paralysis that ruined Aunt Gina's life.

Vacation

So, I was off to my vacation in Spain on the last day of October. My left hand continued acting up. Soon, my index finger curled, too, and nearly every night I woke up from the pain that was shooting and twisting through my hand and forearm. There was also a constant sensation of tingling and numbness in my hand.

The backdrop of scenic Catalonian and Andalusian landscapes made the experience even more surreal. I remember one night in Granada when I woke up from a throbbing pain in my hand and was pacing back and forth in the room, trying to calm down the pain. A silver circle of full moon shone through the window, hanging right above the stark silhouette of the Alhambra. Needless to say, it was not the best way to enjoy the gorgeous view.

During the daytime, my pain was less but still present. I had a hard time picking up my backpack with my left hand or pressing my hand against any flat surface.

By the last day of my vacation, the middle finger on my right hand curled, too. Pain, numbness, and tingling spread to the right hand, and I could not think of anything else, other than what kind of life waited for me if I lost the ability to use both hands.

As I spent many nights awake, I tried to go to The Clinic's website to schedule an appointment with Dr. B, but it didn't

15

work on my mobile phone. I could see that every time I logged on, there were fewer and fewer available appointments, but I could not book one for myself.

At times I wished I could just go home and take care of my health, but I was hopelessly stuck in the schedule and itinerary of my trip. The only thing left for me was to worry. Not being able to spring into action to fix my problems was the worst that could happen to someone of my personality type. I felt trapped.

Downward Spiral

The minute I walked into my house upon return from Spain, I sent a desperate email to my doctor, questioning my carpal tunnel syndrome (CTS) diagnosis and asking for new evaluation.

She, unfortunately, was out for two weeks. Thankfully, another doctor referred me to a neurological evaluation – but I had to wait until the neurology department called me back. After a few days of waiting for their call, I checked in to see why nobody was reaching out to me. Worry not, a nice lady on the phone told me – they will call you back in a few days, just wait.

Waiting proved hard. Every day, I found my condition worsening. The pins and needles became louder, my fingers felt swollen and numb, the nightly bouts of pain more disturbing. I had heard before, but never understood the description of neuropathic pain – until now. It feels like hundreds of fire ants are crawling under your skin. It was the worst pain I'd experienced in my life, because it was so strong and because there was no end to it. I also noticed that my grip in both hands weakened substantially.

In addition, I realized that Reynaud Syndrome, a condition that I have had on and off for many years, became much worse. Reynaud Syndrome is a cardio-vascular condition, causing extremities (fingers, toes, or nose) to get numb and suddenly turn white or even purple. I never considered it a concern before, but now it started progressing at an alarming speed. Per Mayo Clinic's web site "doctors don't completely understand the cause of Reynaud's attacks, but blood vessels in the hands and feet appear to overreact to cold temperatures or stress."

In my case, my middle fingers, already crippled, would suddenly start going completely numb, and then turn white and eventually purple. Pain levels would rise, as if my fingers were screaming for help. The index fingers and ring fingers would often join the show and then I would be rushing to the sink to stick my extremely painful fingers under hot water, hoping that heat would get the blood moving. To avoid pain, I started occasionally wearing gloves, even in 70-degree weather. Before, I did not take Reynaud seriously; it didn't bother me much as it came and went. Now it became debilitating enough that I decided to mention it to Dr. B. as another symptom that didn't fit into the CTS diagnosis.

It is amazing how small things seem to hurt you the most. When one day I got up in the morning and could not slice soft cheese, my spirit was crushed. I broke down and cried, biting from the entire big slab of cheese and wondering which one of my abilities I would lose next. I don't know exactly why not being able to slice cheese was that last straw, but I was terrified. This is where I was: not being able to tie my shoes, use a knife or a fork, or write my signature on a check – and it kept getting worse.

17

I remember the day when I had to start wearing a pair of grip gloves because I could no longer turn the round knob on the front door of my house or hold a steering wheel while driving. Soon, I had to give up driving long distances on a freeway because the pain and numbness became unbearable about 15-20 minutes into driving.

At work, I could no longer take notes in my notepad – my hands refused to cooperate. I could no longer keep my hands on the tabletop during meetings, as raising my hands above my waistline aggravated the pain. My arms had to hang down so I could tolerate the crawling fire ants. Typing became harder and harder. I could not hold my phone in front of my face for more than 30-45 seconds (yes, I timed it!) since my hand would be above my waistline. I had to put the phone down on the table in front of me and use it that way. All these bizarre idiosyncratic symptoms were bewildering and scary. Upon return from Spain, my condition had gone completely off the cliff in just about four weeks.

Whatever little was left of my sense of humor, it could be summarized in one sentence that I used to describe my condition: My middle fingers gave me a middle finger, and so did my hands.

I needed help, desperately. But it was slow to come. Every couple hours I checked my email for the messages from The Clinic, and kept my phone nearby so I would not miss the call from the neurology department. But they were not calling, and my primary doctor did not seem to be interested in seeing me until after the neurological evaluation was done, so I started looking for alternatives.

That's when I went to see a chiropractor.

Before You Move On

I need to ask my reader for some patience here. In the next two chapters, I am going to talk in great details about what happened in the next three months - not to vent, but for a more important reason.

Throughout my ordeal, I heard similar stories from fellow sufferers, stories of wandering through the maze of the healthcare system, confusing diagnoses, unnecessary treatments, excruciating delays, and unwanted addictive painkillers. If you understand that you are not the first one doubting your diagnoses, questioning prescribed treatments, or confused by contradictory symptoms, you may shorten your path to your own recovery.

If you, my reader, or someone you know, are suffering from a chronic neurological condition, whether it is carpal tunnel syndrome, chronic pain, migraines, or dystonia, it may be important for you to read through the details: It may protect you from repeating mistakes made by the newcomers to your medical condition before you. You may find some answers to the questions that you already have. You may feel more assertive questioning your diagnosis and, by doing so, arrive on a better treatment, whether it comes from your doctor or some other source. So, please, stick with my story through Chapter 2 and Chapter 3, no matter how full of unnecessary details and chaotic it may seem. The timeline and events in my story appear chaotic because they reflect my real-life chaotic search for a solution.

But even if you jump over the next two chapters now, make sure to come back to them before making your judgement about the validity of my experience and my conclusions. Like in a grade school math class, I am showing you my work, not just giving you a solution to the problem. Your solution to the problem may be different from mine, but the overall experience of searching for the solution may end up being similar, so give it a try.

Chapter 2. The Maze
Chiropractor Sandy
I had had some good luck with chiropractors before.

A chiropractor helped me out of a sudden, prolonged, severe attack of lower back pain after a fall during a hike in my early 40s.

As I struggled with pain, my primary physician recommended I stop yoga and hiking. She told me: At your age, you need to stop jumping up and down and start taking care of yourself. I was 44. I thanked her, got up, and left her office, never to see her again.

About two years of regular chiropractic adjustments and yoga – and I left my back pain behind and started backpacking in the mountains.

About eight years later, I had an outbreak of Morton's neuroma, a very painful knot in the ball of my foot that made walking even half a mile nearly impossible.

After the orthopedic surgeon prescribed me a $350 pair orthotics (which proved to be completely useless) and suggested a subsequent surgical procedure with an unimpressive success rate of about 60%, I changed the course and went to the chiropractor. Two adjustments – and I was back to my 15-mile hiking regimen. Another few follow-up monthly adjustments – and I haven't heard from my Morton's neuroma since.

So, with full faith in chiropractors, I went to see Sandy, a former civil engineer and a chiropractor in her second career. Her youthful look belied her story that she worked as an engineer for a while and then spent years getting through the school of chiropractic. Her modest office, furnished with miscellaneous shelves and chairs, looked meager compared to The Clinic. I guess that's as much as she could afford as far as decorating her office – but I liked her frugality because my insurance did not cover my visits and I was paying out of my pocket.

I began telling her that I was in pain, that I was losing my hands to the terrifying illness, and I knew in my heart that my doctor was wrong about the diagnosis. There were so many symptoms that didn't match it that I was certain that it was **not** carpal tunnel syndrome, but I had no idea what it was.

Sandy agreed with me. Unlike Dr. B, she did not exude unshakeable confidence that she knew everything. Instead, she asked me some interesting questions: Have you found some body positions that make you feel better? Have you had any stressful experiences prior to developing symptoms? Is your upper back always tight like this?

At that moment, it occurred to me that, indeed, I had a very stressful time both at work and at home in the months prior to the onset of pain. I acknowledged that my upper back had been quite tight and even painful for a while. I demonstrated how I rotated my left arm at the shoulder this way and my right arm at the shoulder another way, to ease the tingling and burning pain at night – and how it worked, albeit temporarily.

She then checked out my upper back, shoulders, neck, and arms, and concluded that all my upper body was a tight knot of stressed muscles and that I had a pinched nerve, very likely in three places: neck, shoulder, and elbow, which was causing symptoms in my hands. She was clearly zeroing in on what had always been my problem area – my upper back and shoulders.

Then she spent 30 minutes massaging and stretching my neck, shoulder, and arm muscles – and I left her office with less pain, less numbness, and almost no tingling. She warned me about potential pain coming my way after this procedure. And, sure enough, I woke up at night with pain everywhere: hands, arms, entire back. But in the morning, I regained a bit of mobility in my wrists and the next night I slept better. She gave me homework to do: stretches and massages with a set of two tennis balls or a foam roller.

Unlike Dr. B, she could see me as often as I needed her. She was compassionate and willing to try different options. Improvements after her adjustment lasted for a few hours, but even a few hours without the fire ants crawling under my skin were a big relief. A few more adjustments – and I was hopeful that the improvements might stick.

But after two weeks of hope, I started getting worse again. My desperation spiked again, so I restarted my search for answers. Looking for information on Google somehow gave me a bit of a mental break. As if understanding my illness could help cure it. While it could not cure me, searching on Google definitely took my desperate mind away from returning endlessly to Aunt Gina and her suffering, but I still could not help but worry about what awaited me in the near future.

Acupressure. The Kathleen

A few years before my ordeal, I started taking acupressure classes. I signed up for the acupressure class nearly by accident. At that time, I did not know that acupressure would open the entire new world to me.

Acupressure is one of the branches of Chinese medicine. It is an ancient cousin, or rather a predecessor, of the much better-known acupuncture, the main difference between the two being that the acupressurist uses hands instead of needles. Oldest known written instructions in acupressure go back thousands of years.

To learn that ailments can be relieved by activating certain points on the surface of the body was, in a way, a continuation of my fascination with chiropractic. Except now I was not a mindless consumer of the art, but rather an apprentice in the practice of it.

My first instructor at the acupressure school was Kathleen. Kathleen, revered by her students and clients, is also known in our local acupressure community as The Kathleen. She is an ultimate healer: intelligent, compassionate, perceptive, and wise. She reads people instantly. Her advice is always offered in a way that would likely be accepted by her client, although it may not be even recognized as such at the first glance.

After a series of chiropractic treatments did not deliver lasting improvement, I reached out to Kathleen. Kathleen identified my condition from the viewpoint of Chinese medicine. And her conclusion could be loosely translated into the Western terms as this: an exhaustion of the nervous system that led to the unusual reaction of my joints and muscles. It was very consistent with my long history of stiffness and pain in my muscles, tight upper back and shoulders, frequent migraines – nothing unusual for my type A personality, which in terms of Chinese medicine is better described as a dominating wood element. In that respect, she

24

was in agreement with Sandy that a stressful experience could be the culprit in my misery.

I left Kathleen's tiny office feeling better. The next day, my symptoms seemed to be almost entirely gone. Repeat session made it stick for a few days. I was excited and hopeful. But not for long.

Results of her treatments, very encouraging at first, faded away a couple of weeks later. Feeling that she probably hit a wall, Kathleen referred me to her friend, acupuncturist K.. I was dismayed that even The Kathleen could not help me, but I was still holding out my hope for Chinese medicine.

Stuck

Meanwhile, all my waking hours outside my work and medical appointments I spent online, reading and learning about CTS. After all, this was a diagnosis that had been handed to me and I needed to figure out how to either accept it or to find a way to debunk it. I was learning a lot.

CTS in the modern world is somehow commonly associated with typing on a computer keyboard. As far as I was concerned, I spent most of my day at work **not** typing. A brief look at my calendar would make one wonder how I would even find time to type! I spent most of my workday in meetings where I hardly used my hands. But even when I typed, I was not a superfast typist. I did what is called 10-key typing, hardly ever looking at the keyboard, but I think as I type, so my pace is rather slow.

As I searched for answers, I could not understand how I developed the symptoms at least two weeks **after** I stopped stressing my hand with a repetitive paint-scraping movement. There was something else that bothered me in the diagnosis that was handed to me by my ever-confident doctor Dr. B. None of the articles that I read mentioned involuntary contraction of the tendons. The contraction of the tendons is **not** a part of the CTS picture. Another mystery that I could not understand was why the symptoms jumped on to the other hand at the time when I was not exerting my wrists and hands. I learned that it was not unusual for the CTS to spread to the other side, but I couldn't find any explanation why it happened in my case during vacation. At times, I felt like I was wandering around a labyrinth, without an exit in sight.

So, there I was in mid-December, perplexed and stuck. Two weeks after my return from Spain, my doctor B. was back, but no, she was not in a hurry to get me into her office again. I got a sense she didn't really know what to do and therefore, she would rather not see me. So, I decided to remind her about my existence and wrote this plea for help:

Dr. *B,*

I am awaiting the nerve conduction study on 12/11. I am quite anxious about how long it is taking to receive actual medical help and advice while both my hands are now impacted. Every night, I wake up from pain (and yes, I use a wrist brace) and spend a couple hours trying to calm down throbbing pain and numbness. Sometimes, I can go back to sleep, but often not, so at best, I get 5-6 hours of poor sleep per day. In the morning, it takes me about 30 minutes of a warmup before I can hold anything in my hands, 45-60 minutes before I can tie shoelaces or drive a car. Driving is high risk because my hands may get numb in the middle of driving, unpredictably. And it is getting progressively worse.

When she finally responded to my desperate emails, this is what she had to offer: "*We could have ortho take a look and perhaps do a steroid injection to help the nerve calm down. Let me know if you would consider this.*"

My reaction was disbelief and anger. Every day, I was losing my abilities to do basic things. My hands were now bright red and swollen. It felt as if fiery ants were crawling under my skin day and night, and there was no way to stop them. I couldn't sleep, I couldn't write, I couldn't cook, I couldn't open a door to my own house without grip gloves – and all my doctor could offer me was to wait for another month before somebody, hopefully, could tell me why I got so sick so fast, and why this weirdness happened to me out of a blue, for no apparent reason. I expected from my doctor at least an explanation of why, in less than two months, without injury or apparent physical impact, I went from being healthy to being disabled.

She didn't have any explanation, but she had steroid shots available. She couldn't explain the cause, but she suggested that I could "perhaps" take steroids – and she left the decision to me, the patient, stressed out, confused, exhausted by relentless pain, sleep deprivation, worries about losing my job and health insurance along with it, to me, increasingly stressed by daily obsessive Google searches on neuropathic pain in a desperate hope to stumble upon a diagnosis that could make sense.

Looking back, I now understand how the gap between my expectation and the health services I was in fact receiving led to the escalation of my stress and worsening of my condition.

I was looking for a competent, compassionate partner who would take me through the path to recovery. I was looking for health care. What I got instead was a waitress of sorts, with what essentially was a menu, a list of treatments to choose from, each one offering little or no hope for a full recovery but rather requiring ongoing treatments, potentially for the rest of my life.

Looking back, I understand that I must be fair to my doctors. At that time, I expected nothing less than a magic pill. I was looking for a miracle that would instantly turn the clock back to the moment when I was healthy. It took me a long time to understand how wrong I was.

But wait! Dr. B. finally offered to see me. In her office, I told her that my pain levels were unbearable. I explained that I had a relatively high tolerance to pain, giving her examples: I did not take painkillers when my four wisdom teeth were removed at once and even after the emergency appendectomy. As a matter of fact, I ended up with a burst appendix exactly because I rated my abdominal pain level at seven out of ten, enough for the nurse on the hotline to decide that it wasn't high enough for appendicitis, so I did not end up in ER for another four days.

As I told Dr. B all the above, I hoped that my story conveyed to her that my pain level was an indication of a true need for help. Smiling and calm as always, she understood that I was in discomfort, but she needed me to follow the standard treatments that were offered for CTS. When I asked her whether her CTS diagnosis could explain my curled finger, she smiled and changed the subject. She said that steroids were a recommended treatment for my diagnosis. Whether the diagnosis was right or wrong did not seem to matter. In short: She couldn't explain my symptoms with her diagnosis, but I had to follow the standard treatment for the diagnosis. She assured me that if steroids did not help, we could always go for surgery. As I was leaving her office, she was all smiles and confidence. She told me to hang in there until the electromyography test. However, I was not good at following her advice.

Here is my next email to Dr. B:

Neurology dept called me today to reschedule the test again. I feel powerless and neglected. I wish I went to other practitioners before my condition progressed so far that I can barely hold onto my job.

I think The Clinic lives on a clock that is very different from the one of their patients. I watch my energy draining away and myself heading to a disability at a very fast speed. However, The Clinic is not in a hurry. I can still type, thank God. But I can no longer handwrite. I get by on 4-5 hours of sleep and can barely function at work. I am learning a lot about peripheral neuropathy (this is my working hypothesis until proved otherwise) and there are treatments available. For The Clinic, I still have carpal tunnel in left hand, so I was given two recommendations so far: use a brace at night and have steroid shots to ease the pain. Should other options be offered to me? some are cheap, like acupuncture or PT [physical therapy].

I got no response for a few days. Apparently, my rapidly approaching disability was no concern to Dr. B. I continued my descent into the downward spiral.

Nerves Are Very Logical

The wheels of a managed healthcare system turn slowly. Seven weeks after my return from Spain, I was finally able to see a neurologist for the electromyography (EMG) test. By then, my condition was much worse. Both Sandy and Kathleen could not succeed in curing my illness. I was terrified by how quickly I went from being an energetic, physically active, and generally healthy person to a complete cripple in just under two months, without any precipitating injury or a noticeable trigger of any kind. I kept thinking of Aunt Gina who took years to get to this degree of incapacitation. How bad was it going to be for me in the future?

Nervous as if I was taking a test for the chance to live, I appeared in front of Dr. W., a neurologist. He was a mild-mannered man in his 60s. He apologized that he could not see me sooner due to the overload of work in his department.

He warned me that this procedure could be painful because he would be running electric signals through my hands. He put sensors on my hands and turned the device on. When the procedure was over, I laughed and told him that the pain from his device was nothing compared to the daily torture that I went through all the time, especially at night.

We then discussed the results. He concluded that signal degradation in both my hands indicated definite nerve damage and recommended that I undergo a steroid injection and, if that did not help, surgery. At that point, I asked him whether either of the two procedures would fix my curled fingers. He did his best to avoid the answer. He could see that I was very skeptical about the CTS diagnosis, that I was upset that it took so long for The Clinic to have me scheduled for the procedure, and, despite my allocated time being only 30 minutes, he offered to give me a consultation beyond the basic EMG procedure. I was floored. I was finally seeing a doctor who was willing to discuss my illness. Unlike Dr B, he did not repeatedly state that I had CTS and because I had CTS and that I had to go through steroid injections because that's what was recommended for CTS.

Dr. W was a nice man. He definitely loved his craft. He walked out of the room and came back with a big, heavy book on neurology. He also brought a brochure on CTS, written and published sometime in the '40s or '50s. He told me that to him this brochure was still the best material on CTS because it was so clearly written. He started with the explanation of why he chose neurology some 40 years ago. He was a very analytical person and when he was in medical school at UCLA, he found nerves to be very logical. He showed me the diagrams and drawings in the book. The electrical signals that power our nervous system either exist or not. That's why it is so logical – here he got excited. You see – he pointed at my chart – both of your hands show significant degradation in the strength of electrical signal. That's why you feel the pain, numbness, and tingling because there is simply not enough electricity to feed the tendons.

That's when I asked him again about my curled fingers. How does the degradation of electrical signal explain the fact that I can't straighten out my fingers? How confident are you in the CTS diagnosis? - I asked. He said, 75%. I asked him, what about the other 25%? He insisted that 75 was still greater than 25. To that, I had to agree – his math sounded very logical.

Leaving the logic of the other 25% aside, I asked him about the effectiveness of the steroid injection procedure and the rate of success. He looked puzzled. You know – he said – I used to run a clinic with my partner, a hand surgeon. When I referred people to my partner, they would come back to me and I would evaluate them after the procedure. But that was a long time ago. Now at The Clinic, I just refer people out, but I don't see them after the treatment. They go for the follow-up to their primary doctors. That was a good question, he said.

As we progressed into our conversation about the logical nature of the nervous system, he remembered a patient who he'd seen some years back. The patient had a bad case of CTS in one hand, but Dr. W did EMG on both hands. The hand with no pain at all had a much deeper degradation of electrical signals. I can't recall where the conversation went after that point. I think I quickly agreed that nerves were very logical and got ready to leave.

We parted ways as friends. We talked about our kids and how proud we were of them, about our professional fields, and about the logic of neurology. I really liked him. I thanked him for the attention and extra time he gave me. I believe that he even mentioned the word "dystonia," which became so important to me later, but it didn't catch my attention at that time.

But I still didn't have the answer to my question about my curled fingers. My curled fingers didn't fit into the logic of the nervous system. At least, into Dr. W's logic.

Second Opinion
Of course, when I got home, I went for a second opinion. I consulted with Dr. Google who knew everything, almost as

much as Dr B. Judging by how much time Dr. B spent on her computer during my visits, I hoped that she would be familiar with Dr. Google's opinion, too.

Dr. Google, on behalf of various medical experts, had a lot to say on carpal tunnel syndrome. Some of it spoke in favor of a surgery.

"In summary, existing long-term outcomes research generally indicates that OCTR (Open Carpal Tunnel Release) is an effective long-term treatment method. Clinical success is shown to occur at a rate of 75–90 %" [1]

But Dr. Google also had some negative things to say about surgery, so it was a mixed bag:

"recurrence is reported in 4–57 % of cases" [1]

This is what I found on the subject of surgery on the National Institute of Health's site: "fewer than half of individuals report their hand(s) feeling completely normal following surgery. Some residual numbness or weakness is common." [2]

I also learned from the same National Institute of Health, that effectiveness of steroid injection for CTS was studied with the following results:

- Symptoms improved on their own in about 30 out of 100 people (placebo injections)
- Symptoms improved after corticosteroids were injected in about 75 out of 100 people.
- In other words, the treatment provided noticeable short-term relief from symptoms in about 45 out of 100 people. [3]

Just think about it. You are about to get a service from a vendor.

The vendor offers you two options: service A, a one-time deal, which statistically has less than 50% full success rate or a recurring service B with a statistical success rate of 45% that must be repeated three - four times a year, with possible negative consequences for you (side effects). Or you can use no service at all and you have one chance out of three that your problem may disappear by itself. Even if your cost is next to nothing, would you hire this vendor if they were a plumber or a general contractor?

I could not accept either one of those outcomes, especially because nobody so far could explain my curled fingers. It was not even excruciating pain. It was the mystery of what made my muscles contract without any rhyme or reason to it that consumed my mind.

The image of Aunt Gina progressively crippled by incurable illness was always with me. I was scared. The more I was scared, the more aggressively I searched for answers and help. I was too scared to give up.

Against the Brick Wall
As I was trying to get to the bottom of my diagnosis, I also wanted to get a treatment, but not the steroid injection, which seemed more like a gamble to me. One thing I was certain about: I definitely did not want to visit my always-confident Dr. B. However, I didn't know whether another doctor would be any better. At least Dr. B had some history on me and, hopefully, some sense of responsibility to the patient she had been seeing for three years.

Since Sandy's exercises seemed to ease my pain at least temporarily, I asked for a referral to physical therapy. Sandy's visits were not covered by my insurance, so I wanted to get at least some help from The Clinic, which would only cost me a $15 copay. But Dr. B didn't respond to my request for a referral to physical therapy. I was in too much pain and frustration to even send her a reminder. I was close to being done with her.

A week after the visit to the neurologist, Dr. W, as I diligently searched The Clinic's website, I discovered that they had something called a pain management clinic. I asked Dr. B for a referral to the pain management clinic, explaining that after eight weeks of excruciating neuropathic pain, I was exhausted. I needed help. Looks like Dr. B would have given me anything, as long as it was not what I was asking for:

The pain management program is really to help treat chronic pain that hasn't responded to our standard treatments. I would recommend we start with having you evaluated by the hand specialist and PT, as these are our first line treatments, and I do think we can help you. If you need something in the interim for pain I can certainly help with that (i.e. An anti-inflammatory like Aleve or relafen, or narcotic like tramadol)

So, now she was interested in offering me PT (physical therapy). Maybe Dr. B had a plan, simply because she "knows better." But this is how her plan looked from my perspective:

- Ignore the patient's complaints for a while
- Put the patient on the treatment (steroids) that the patient, concerned with the possible side effects, resents

- Ignore patient's requests for any treatments other than steroids
- Give the patient an opioid tramadol
- Two months after the initial complaint, give the patient the "first line treatment," which the patient has been asking for in the first place.
- Deny the patient a referral to the pain management clinic and make the patient go through another few months of pain and disability to get the patient to a chronic state.

I was angry at Dr. B, but I was elated that I had at last wrestled a referral to PT from her hands.

That was the last time I spoke to Dr. B.

Meanwhile, I got an appointment with the hand surgeon in less than three weeks, almost nothing compared to the eight weeks of neuropathic pain. The wheels of managed care started turning.

Physical Therapy

I was excited about the prospects of physical therapy. After all, Sandy's foam roller and two balls in a mesh bag eased my pain. The Kathleen also recommended a well-used tennis ball to put under my back, right under the painful spots. Both things really helped, although temporarily. It gave me some hope that if not the muscle contractures, at least the pain can be helped by PT.

But there was an obstacle: When I called to schedule an appointment, I was told that I had to take a class on repetitive stress injury (RSI) first. The next class was in five weeks. I went ballistic. I asked to speak with the head of the PT department. I was prepared to fight the brick wall again. But a miracle happened.

The head of the PT department picked up the phone. She understood my situation. She understood that waiting for five more weeks would be too much. She understood that I likely did not have a repetitive stress injury. She also felt a lot of stress in my voice. She waived the class requirement, and I could now appear in front of a physical therapist. I couldn't believe my luck. I kept thanking her and literally couldn't stop. I loved the physical therapy department already. I was hopeful.

Leigh, my PT, was a petite, slim woman. She had a dry sense of humor. She was fast, energetic, and spoke in short, forceful sentences. She pulled out a protractor and measured the angles at which my wrists bent. My wrists were never very flexible before, but now they barely bent outwards. They did not look good. Wasting no time, Leigh got to work. She packed every minute of my appointment with action: She identified my problem areas, she walked me through my homework, and even found a few minutes at the end to give me a relaxing massage. She would have loved to see me every week, but unfortunately, her calendar booked fast and she was only allowed to schedule one appointment at a time. Her next available appointment was in two weeks. Still, I left her office relieved. Her warm, compassionate, and forceful presence gave me hope.

I went home with the homework from Leigh, which I did religiously. I did even more than she wanted me to do, despite the pain and stiff resistance of my hands and wrists. I did Leigh's exercises and Sandy's exercises. I wanted to get well. Working hard on my exercises through pain and struggle somehow brought me a sense of purpose and peace. However, the relief from pain was rather minor and temporary, and none of the exercises seemed to uncurl my fingers.

Acupuncture

Meanwhile, I was still seeing The Kathleen. After each session, I saw a reduction in the night-time excruciating pain. But then the pain slowly rose again, with tingling and numbness continuing. What concerned me the most was that my hands were still curled. The homework from Leigh and Sandy also helped only temporarily.

Time to try another practitioner, Kathleen's friend K. K.'s office was a place that you wouldn't want to leave. Every room had beautiful plants, Chinese watercolors, little water fountains, and soft thick rugs. K. himself was all attention and kindness. His diagnosis was also consistent with Kathleen's. He thought that he could rid me of pain in about ten sessions. He put me on the table and stuck needles in me. After he was done with regular needles, he turned on a laser machine and did acupuncture in the 21st-century way. He sent me home with three bottles of herbs and warned that I may be a bit tired that day and the day after. He was wrong: I was completely exhausted for two and half days, but then I found myself on a slow but steady upswing for the following week.

The numbness and tingling subsided and so did the tightness in my shoulders, neck, and wrists. I started slowly regaining mobility in my wrists. My fingers were still crippled and painful, but they seemed to move slightly better. I started restoring my yoga practice. I was elated. K. gave me herbs for better sleep, and I started sleeping a bit better.

However, about ten days after the first treatment, my hands started swelling even more. The pain level rose again, and over-the-counter painkillers did not work anymore. My sleep deteriorated. I remembered what Leigh told me about Epsom salt soak to reduce swelling and pain. I started spending thirty minutes before work and in the evening soaking my hands in warm water with Epsom salt. It eased the pain for a couple of hours. A friend told me about Voltaren (Diclofenac), a topical pain reliever. Of course, it was not covered by my insurance, but $80 out-of-pocket seemed a low price to pay for couple hours of relief per day. I later found Topricin, a homeopathic cream that worked even better and was much cheaper. I stocked up on Topricin: one tube at work, one tube at home, one tube in the purse. There were days when I had to apply it every thirty minutes.

This is where I was by the end of January 2016. I now slept in the upright position, seated on the couch, because my arms must be hanging down, otherwise, the pain would not let me sleep. I could no longer hold my small mobile phone in front of me as I read – my hands started tingling and pain levels rose after less than one minute. Books were out of the question – I couldn't hold them, but I couldn't read anything anyway because of the brain fog. My hands were red, swollen, and extremely sensitive to cold. I had to wear gloves in the produce section of the supermarket because touching apples or oranges with bare hands made my pain unbearable and triggered a Reynaud's syndrome attack. I regretted purchasing my usual season subscription to the symphony since I couldn't sit in the chair with my hands resting in my lap for forty minutes straight, even with Voltaren generously lathered on my hands. Music, until recently one of the main joys of my life, was no longer a joy.

Meanwhile, K. was working hard. I ended up with more and more bottles of herbs. I saw him twice a week now. He put me on a very restrictive diet to reduce swelling, and it seemed to be working.

One day, K. told me that he reached out to his teacher and got some good advice on my condition. He explained that his teacher was a top acupuncturist in the country. He probably wanted to reassure me that I was in good hands, but what I sensed was just the opposite. I now believed that he was running out of his options. He was optimistic that he got some good recommendations from his very experienced teacher. He needed to alter his treatment and add more herbs, and I should see improvement shortly. But another couple of weeks went by, and I still saw only minor reduction in the pain while my fingers seemed to be curled even more. I now took ten - twelve pills up to six times a day. Some of them had to be taken with meals, some in between meals, and meals themselves were almost like pills since I was not allowed to eat what I liked. All of the above made my head spin and filled my life with even more stress.

I slept better with his herbs, but keeping up with the restrictive diet, taking herbs four - six times a day, along with Sandy/Leigh exercises, Epsom salt hand soak, twice a week visits to K., and at least once a week visits to various The Clinic's doctors became overwhelming.

I still had to go to work every day - and it was my key to the health insurance, and, of course, the only way I could have income. If I didn't work – I couldn't afford health care. Worries about being able to keep my job continued to grow as my medical bills mounted. And my condition was not, by any means, encouraging.

I wondered now how Aunt Gina managed to maintain her always-optimistic demeanor in the face of the all-consuming illness.

Lifeline

I was very lucky to have a fairly secure job with good benefits. A typical Type A personality, I put my heart and soul into my work and have a reputation as a diligent worker and a strong performer.

A manager in the IT department, I spent at least half of my work time in meetings, so my job did not require much typing or direct computer work. I had to type, depending on a day, anywhere from a few dozen email messages to half a dozen pages of documents. This was why I found the entire concept of repetitive stress injury and carpal tunnel diagnosis absolutely not applicable to me. The stress of my work was not on my hands. The stress of my work was on my nerves.

There is a lot of pressure in the fast-moving IT environment. Usually, my day was packed with projects, deadlines, emergencies - and I could hardly find time for a lunch break. Often, I had to work extra hours. I used to get dehydrated at work because I never had time to get up and make myself a cup of tea - until I bought a tea kettle and kept it on my desk so I could make tea while working. Steady stream of questions, daily crises that need my attention, conflicts between various people and groups needing my involvement - all but guaranteed that by the end of the day I often felt like I had just been pulled out of a pressure cooker.

So, there I was in January 2016. After those three excruciatingly long months that I had been living with unending pain and loss of dexterity in my hands, I was no longer on top of my game. I had a hard time typing and therefore I was behind on writing up large documents; I couldn't reply to all the emails that needed my response. Being a perfectionist, I was frustrated. Whenever I could substitute email with personal appearance, I did that. But often I still needed to type. So, I lathered Topricin on my hands, waited for few minutes for the pain to start receding, and then got to work.

What made matters worse was that I had to keep my arms hanging down, otherwise, neuropathic ants under my skin got more and more agitated and their sting became unbearable. So, I typed and then rested.

I suffered little embarrassments in the workplace. I remember a day when an employee walked in with a document he needed me to sign – and I could not do it because my pain and swelling were so bad at the moment that I could not scribble my name, date, and my very short signature. I had to come up with a lame excuse why I could not do it immediately. Once he left, I had to close the door and practice a few times before I could finally produce something legible. By the end of that exercise, I was exhausted.

There were a few occasions when I didn't have my grip gloves with me. It took some creativity to come up with a good explanation why I was hanging out in front of the door with a round knob, waiting for the next person to come and open it for me.

Instead of responding to emails, I would walk over to people's desks and talk to them in person. They often wondered why I chose to come by three times instead of sending them a message.

In the meeting rooms, I was always looking for a chair in the back row, to hide behind others and let my arms hang instead of putting my hands on the table or in my lap.

I didn't want to attract attention to my new strange habits. Which, of course, added more stress to my already-stressful situation. I asked to remove the armrest from my chair to allow my arms to hang when I was not typing. I carried Topricin with me at all times. I was struggling, with no end in sight. My mind was not as sharp anymore. I had a hard time concentrating and thinking things through.

I asked HR to schedule an ergonomic evaluation of my workstation, which my employer offered. Unfortunately, it took weeks for the occupational therapist to arrive and another few weeks, if not months, for the equipment to be installed. The demand for ergonomic adjustment was high in the office as quite a few people, some of them young, suffered from back, neck or wrist pain. I find it interesting that our sit-at-a-desk jobs are so demanding physically that our backs, necks, and hands start falling apart by the age of 25-30. I wonder how the people of pre-knowledge era managed to dig trenches, plow fields, march as soldiers for miles with heavy packs - and still get years of mileage out of their bodies.

So, I was quite worried whether I could keep up with the demands of my job. It was my greatest luck that those three months of December 2015 – February 2016 were a slow time between big projects. My mental fog, my exhaustion, and frequent medical appointments probably were not too visible as I didn't have to navigate too many complex and challenging decisions or be available more than 40 hours per week. Yet, gradually I realized that I was falling behind.

After a long hesitation, I confessed to my boss that I was having some health problems, and I would have to take a lot of time off and would not be as productive as I used to be. Having a reputation for being a diligent and responsible worker helped. My boss was very supportive and willing to cut me some slack while I was recovering. I could not bring myself to reveal that I doubted whether my recovery was even possible. Still, knowing that I had backing and understanding from my superiors helped in a short run, as I was juggling three - four medical appointments every week, mostly during my office hours.

I started delegating more of the tasks that I used to do myself to my team. They were good people. They didn't mind, whether they noticed anything wrong with me or not. Still, as my ability to take notes in the meetings, to respond to the emails, to write documents continued to deteriorate, as my mental fog became thicker, I started giving serious consideration to what to do if I didn't recover soon and had to go on disability and eventually stop working.

But, despite all the challenges that I faced in the office, my job became my lifeline. The structure it created in my life, the need to get out of bed every morning held me together. When I was working, in my own mind I was a worthy human being. I was afraid to fall off the bandwagon. I was afraid of even discussing a short-term disability because I knew that once on disability, I may not be able to return to working. Something inside me resisted the idea of disability so fiercely that for a moment I wondered if I needed to see a therapist who would talk me into starting the disability process. I have never been on disability before, and going through the bureaucratic process stressed me out more than showing up to work every day and putting on a happy face.

Despite the worries, I held on to my job even at the times when I felt it was impossible to get up in the morning and go to work. As hard as it was, every day I put a smile on my face the best I could and went to work, powered by the fear of losing a job and a stubborn determination that I could not explain even to myself - no matter what.

Chapter 3. Rock Bottom
The Wall Is Getting Taller and Denser
As time went by, I still didn't know the diagnosis. Since Sandy, Kathleen, and K. did not cure me in two months, I doubted their conclusions. They all seemed puzzled and not sure how to help me. The more puzzled they were, the more worried I was. Having come full circle, I pinned my last hope on The Clinic's doctors, equipped with MRI and other sophisticated devices. I knew I must find the answer.

Around the second half of January, I went to see the hand surgeon, Dr. S. He was supposed to determine whether I needed a steroid injection or surgery, but I hoped that he would challenge the diagnosis of CTS – there ought to be somebody with a medical degree who would be willing to consider symptoms that did not fit the standard schema. He asked me to sit down and started looking at my X-Ray and MRI. He took time, he did not speak, he seemed to be puzzled by what he saw. I waited patiently as he carefully and diligently examined my records, my MRI, my X-ray. I began hoping that he was that miracle doctor who would dismiss the CTS diagnosis and explain what was wrong with me.

I expected just about anything, but not what he said when he finally started speaking. He told me that he could give me a steroid injection and if the steroid injection did not work, surgery was another possibility. He then explained that the steroid injection may not last long and I might have to return for more injections. He also talked about how the surgery was going to be done and what to expect after surgery. He was 100% on board with the CTS diagnosis.

I was so stunned that I thanked him and went home, questioning my own sanity. If everybody told me that what I had was a trivial CTS, I'd better agree. I was beginning to seriously consider surrendering to the steroid injection.

Meanwhile, I finally had a new primary doctor, Dr. P. It took me a while to find her. Since I had learned my lesson, I tried to find a doctor for whom reviews had been posted online. The Clinic did not have reviews for their doctors on their website, but some of the doctors worked elsewhere before joining The Clinic, like Dr. P.

Dr. P had some very heartwarming reviews, but she wasn't accepting new patients at that time. I learned my ways around the world of managed care and realized that there were some wonderful people who worked the clerical desks at The Clinic – they could do a lot for the patients, we just needed to know how to ask. I called member services and a very nice lady promised to put me on the wait list. A few weeks later, she called me back and signed me up.

Dr. P. greeted me with a warm smile. She was compassionate and wanted to help. Unfortunately, she seemed to be quite puzzled by my symptoms. It soon became clear to me that neurology was not her forte, so I couldn't really expect to break through the wall of CTS diagnosis with her. But when I mentioned to her that Dr. B denied my request for a referral to the pain management clinic, she instantly said: "We don't want you to be in pain for six months to get help" and – a miracle! – I had a referral to the pain management clinic. It was still few weeks before I could get in, but one month was so much better than six! I will never forget the surge of warm feelings toward Dr. P and sense of relief that I was being helped.

47

Another sign of an attentive physician: Dr. P was concerned with Reynaud's. She wanted to make sure that there was no rheumatoid arthritis in play, and she referred me to the rheumatologist and cardio-vascular specialist.

Downward Spiral Continues

After about six weeks of visits to the acupuncturist K. and generous applications of Topricin, the pain and swelling seemed to subside to more tolerable levels, but my hands were getting more and more limited in range of motion. I still could not straighten my fingers out, and in addition, I now had a hard time bending my fingers. I could no longer make a fist, initially for several morning hours; eventually my hands refused to cooperate for the entire day.

After a while, K. suggested that, in addition to his treatment, maybe I should resume sessions with Kathleen and/or Sandy, to have a massage for my hands and arms. I took K.'s suggestion as a signal that he was not sure what to do. My fear rose to the highest levels. My mind raced through the memories of Aunt Gina, concerns of how I was going to hold on to my job and how I was going to have access to healthcare when I lost my job.

It was early February. It had been less than five months since the day I found my left forearm swollen, but it seemed like an eternity already. Aside from constant pain, my symptoms evolved from weird to outright bizarre. One night, my friend and I were sitting at the dinner table and I noticed that red blotches on my hands start moving. Astonished, we both watched, for at least fifteen - twenty minutes, the bright red blotches moving quite quickly around my hands, while my hands remained motionless on the table. If I didn't have a witness to this color show, I would have thought that I was hallucinating.

Meanwhile, as contractions of my fingers became more and more pronounced, I decided to send a message to the hand surgeon. Here it is:

Dr. S,

During my visit, you mentioned that some of my symptoms are not consistent with CTS and may indicate something else. Can you clarify whether the following symptoms are not typical for CTS:

1. Extreme sensitivity to cold and increase in Reynaud's-type pain attacks in hands
2. Loss of range of motion in wrists
3. Bent and crippled fingers, I cannot straighten them out
4. I noticed that tingling disappears when my arms and hands hang down and increases when my arms are bent in the elbows and hands are above waist level.
5. I do not see any correlation between bending wrists and increase in tingling/pain

He responds the same day:

They are not typical for carpal tunnel syndrome. I am reviewing your case.

It was my first victory against the wall. It was not CTS. But what was it?

Hope Crashed

As I shuttled between K., Sandy, Kathleen, Leigh, neurologist, hand surgeon, cardio-vascular specialist who found me in perfect health as far as his area was concerned, one day Leigh mentioned in passing that she thought she knew what I had.

As I almost jumped out of my chair, she made a disclaimer that I should not take it as a firm diagnosis, but she'd had patients with similar symptoms. What she thought I had was called Complex Regional Pain Syndrome. I told her that it was good news to have a diagnosis. She did not disagree with me that it was better to have a diagnosis than not, but she was doubtful that CRPS is a diagnosis I should feel elated about.

When I got home after my physiotherapy session, I went online and soon started agreeing with Leigh. Yes, my mysterious and weird symptoms seemed to match the definition of Complex Regional Pain Syndrome (CRPS). It was also known by its previous name, Reflex Sympathetic Dystrophy or RSD. The word "dystrophy" alone terrified me. I understood why doctors decided to rename it and give it a name that hides the horror of dystrophic deterioration behind lengthy and boredom-inducing verbiage.

I started with Wikipedia's detailed article on CRPS/RSD. It sported two photos of arms and hands damaged by CRPS. The wrists and hands looked like red balloons and clearly indicated the direction in which my own hands were rapidly moving. One of the photos presented me with a very familiar picture of Aunt Gina's hand. The hand was swollen and clenched. It clearly could not open. The only difference was that Aunt Gina didn't seem to have swelling in her limbs. But I did.

After reading about CRPS for a while, I came to a scary conclusion that it was just one of the buckets in which doctors put symptoms that they simply don't know what to do about. Even doctors seem to be completely perplexed, not only by the nature of the illness but also by the triggers that cause it. They didn't know what caused the onset and why in some rare cases it went away by itself. However, it was more likely to spread to other parts of the body than to heal spontaneously. Sometimes it fully engulfed the entire body. Sometimes, it could be traced to a precipitating injury like a fracture of a limb, but often there seemed to be no obvious cause.

Somewhere, I found stats that put chances of recovery in adults at about 20%. None of the known treatments seemed to offer full recovery. Remission seemed to be somewhat random and mostly temporary.

I started wondering if it would have been better for me to not know what my diagnosis is because my diagnosis offered me very little hope. I now understood what was that atypical Parkinson's that destroyed Aunt Gina. It was CRPS, or RSD as it was known back in those days. But her CRPS did not strike alone. It came with another illness, dystonia. Dystonia (involuntary contraction of the muscles) can be one of the symptoms of CRPS, but it can also happen on its own. And, as far as I could tell from consulting with Dr. Google, both CRPS and dystonia were considered incurable by the official medical community.

Here are some quotes from reputable sources that I didn't find particularly encouraging:

"Currently, there are no medications or treatments to prevent dystonia or slow its progression, nor is there a cure". [4]

"There's no known cure for complex regional pain syndrome (CRPS), but a combination of physical treatments, medication and psychological support can help manage the symptoms." [5]

As I started digging deeper into the medical literature describing successful procedures to help with dystonia, I found that there were some very specific variations of dystonia that could be helped by medications (like Botox), but the list of side effects scared me. To make matters worse, I didn't see any evidence of widespread clinical studies to validate a generalized use of those medications or prove that remission could be permanent. I also got lost in the convoluted classification of various types of dystonia and my head started spinning. There were discussions about nerve blocks, deep brain stimulation (brain implant), peripheral denervation – and my imagination went into overdrive once I realized that denervation meant a destruction of the nerves as the most effective way to stop the pain. [6]

As I feverishly navigated the confusing and often ambiguous online repositories of CRPS information, I pieced together my self-diagnosis. I didn't seem to have a precipitating injury, unless scraping paint with a hand scraper counted as injury. I had swelling, extreme sensitivity to cold and touch, skin on the sides of my fingers felt thin like old parchment, my hands were hot and red as if I had just boiled them, and there were white blotches on them that travelled around in weird patterns. Add neuropathic pain and dystonia – that involuntary contraction of my tendons and ligaments. Nothing matched my symptoms better than descriptions of CRPS, although those appeared to be somewhat varied from one medical site to another.

I was now confident that my carpal tunnel syndrome diagnosis was a product of Dr. B's ignorance about CRPS. However, Dr. B was far from alone in misdiagnosing CRPS. As I learned, most CRPS patients do not get diagnosed properly for a very long time. Instead, they are ping-ponged through the healthcare system, often without a diagnosis, but sometimes with wrong diagnoses.

In my opinion, a wrong diagnosis is much worse than none. Wrong diagnosis sets already very miserable people on the path of useless and often very expensive treatments and ends up making their conditions even more debilitating. When they are finally diagnosed with CRPS, often years later, they are told that any delay in CRPS diagnosis beyond the first three months after the onset significantly reduces the chances of recovery.

Anger boiled inside me, anger at Dr. B and her unshakeable confidence that she was the only one with the knowledge, while her patients were just silent objects who must follow her directives. My sleep was now completely ruined. I woke up from nightmares after one - two hours of shaky sleep and couldn't go back to it, despite the hearty doses of K.'s pills.

My hope was crushed by the 80% probability that I would never recover, that more likely I would get worse. I now noticed what I ignored for a while – that my feet, my ankles, and my knees ad been showing similar signs of tension and pain. Those symptoms had not been strong enough to make me worried. Or, maybe, they would have been strong enough to make me worried – if I hadn't had a much bigger problem at hand – literally, at both hands. But now I knew that CRPS could spread, and I realized that my knees and ankles were sending me another signal of danger.

I told K. about my suspected diagnosis. He seemed to know about CRPS/RDS. He had treated many people with chronic pain, and he assured me that he would get it under control. But weeks went by and my dystonia only got worse. I could no longer drive more than a couple miles without stopping and resting. It appeared that driving faster than 30-35 miles per hour greatly aggravated both neuropathic pain and dystonia. Even grip gloves did not help me to hold on to the steering wheel. Not driving on a freeway made it very hard to get around in my metropolitan area.

But that was not the worst of my problems. I could barely use my hands, and my arms were getting weaker; I was exhausted by pain, medical appointments, the strict diet that K. put me on, and my inability to cook even the most basic meals. I used to love my morning shower, but now I hated it because it caused me even more pain. I tried not to skip showers on weekdays, but it took a lot of will power to do it. I was just a complete wreck.

Diagnosis

I brought up CRPS with Dr. P. She was reluctant to wander into unfamiliar territory. She suggested that I not jump to conclusions until the pain management clinic and rheumatologist completed their evaluation. She was also talking to the hand surgeon Dr. S. They both asked me to be patient.

Being patient is not my strongest suit. I was now a fixture on the web site of NINDS – National Institute of Neurological Disorders, part of National Institute of Health. It kept me both informed and busy. I learned a lot about CRPS. I joined a couple of online forums for people with CRPS and other neurological disorders.

I was on a quest to get an official diagnosis and start the right treatment – if there was any. I was almost paranoid that I was well past the three-month point after the onset of CRPS - which, per medical gurus, is when recovery becomes much more problematic. I learned that CRPS is one of the most misdiagnosed conditions, partly because it is deemed to be a rare disease, but also because most of the symptoms overlap with other neurological diseases and can be very confusing. The more I learned about CRPS, the more I understood why doctors at The Clinic were reluctant to change my original diagnosis no matter how little my condition by now resembled carpal tunnel syndrome.

As my education continued, I learn that in 2003, a closed workshop was held by the world's experts in CRPS to clarify the CRPS diagnostic criteria. My best guess was that it was a closed event and results were not published until 2007 for a very simple reason: The CRPS medical community was debating how to quickly and reliably diagnose a debilitating and stubborn disease that evaded researchers and clinicians for so long. What they published is now called Budapest Protocol or Budapest Criteria.

The excerpt below is sourced from Medscape [7], a subsidiary of WebMD, but is easily available from other sites.

"A clinical diagnosis of CRPS can be made when the following criteria are met:
1. Continuing pain that is disproportionate to any inciting event
2. At least 1 symptom reported in at least 3 of the following categories:
    o Sensory: Hyperesthesia or allodynia

- Vasomotor: Temperature asymmetry, skin color changes, skin color asymmetry
- Sudomotor/edema: Edema, sweating changes, or sweating asymmetry
- Motor/trophic: Decreased range of motion, motor dysfunction (e.g., weakness, tremor, dystonia), or trophic changes (e.g., hair, nail, skin)
3. At least 1 sign at time of evaluation in at least 2 of the following categories:
   - Sensory: Evidence of hyperalgesia (to pinprick), allodynia (to light touch, temperature sensation, deep somatic pressure, or joint movement)
   - Vasomotor: Evidence of temperature asymmetry (>1°C), skin color changes or asymmetry
   - Sudomotor/edema: Evidence of edema, sweating changes, or sweating asymmetry
   - Motor/trophic: Evidence of decreased range of motion, motor dysfunction (e.g., weakness, tremor, dystonia), or trophic changes (e.g., hair, nail, skin)
4. No other diagnosis better explaining the signs and symptoms."

My checklist was easy to fill out:

- I had a continuing pain that was disproportionate to any inciting event. (In my case, the only suspect was scraping the paint for total of about two hours over a course of a few days.)
- I had symptoms in all four categories: sensory (sensitivity to cold and touch), vasomotor (Raynaud Syndrome), sudomotor/edema (extensive swelling), motor/trophic (dystonia).
- I had signs at the time of numerous medication evaluations in all four above categories

- I did not have any other diagnosis better explaining the signs and symptoms.

One of the reasons for the Budapest Protocol, per its authors, was to create a simple yet reliable diagnostic tool, available to primary care physicians, so patients would be directed to the specialists sooner and therefore receive proper treatment during the critical initial phase of the disease. I was convinced that based on the Budapest Protocol, I had CRPS. My doctors, however, were reluctant to agree.

I finally visited the rheumatologist. She, like other doctors before her, was not ready to give up the CTS diagnosis. However, she sent me to have a battery of blood tests done and found no bio markers of arthritis. When I asked her about CRPS, the best she could do was, without much ado, refer me for the full-body bone scan, which can detect changes in the bones caused by a prolonged CRPS condition.

A bone scan is as high-tech as it can get: It is done by a Gamma Camera after a radioactive substance is injected intravenously. The entire event, from the moment of injection, may take up to four - five hours. As I read about it, I learned that since its introduction in the 1970s, the test was re-evaluated for its efficacy in CRPS diagnosis and at least one article on the NIH site [8] noted that "the clinical usefulness of BS remains controversial."

For a couple of days, I am almost inclined to take the test. But, since my CRPS is about four - five months old, my bones are likely intact, so the test may not reveal anything. After some hesitation, I ultimately decided that it would do me little good while at the same time would be too much stress for me to handle.

I remember vividly my emotional state at that moment: knowing about the Budapest Protocol already but lacking confidence and energy to push for it. I grew quite angry that it was much easier to get a referral for a very expensive and useless test than a decisive diagnosis based on a simple checklist.

I decided to wait. I don't remember exactly what I was going to wait for, but I ended up never scheduling the bone test or seeing that rheumatologist again.

Chapter 4. Awakening

Fateful Day

Other than being a Valentine's Day, February 14, 2016 was just another grim day. Exhausted by pain, dystonia, insomnia, restrictive diet, pills, procedures, I make an appointment with The Kathleen. I hoped for some temporary relief from my miseries and, even more so for a decent night of sleep after her session. As her hands moved around my body and I started to relax a little bit, we talked. As much as I appreciated her acupressure treatments, our conversation was an equally valuable part of the session. It revolved around my specific health problems, but the subject easily moved to the general topics and, as always, I appreciated Kathleen's wit and wisdom. She was one of the best psychotherapists that I knew, although her therapy was just a free bonus added to every conversation that I had with her. Her advice was always offered as a suggestion, but over the years, I came to the realization that I'd better listen to her in-between-the-lines suggestions. She briefly mentioned John Sarno, a doctor from New York, who had an almost cult-like following for treating difficult cases of chronic back pain. Not ready to recognize the advice disguised as a suggestion, I promptly pointed out that my problem area was not my back but rather everything except my back. She responded that apparently his method worked on other types of chronic pain. I vaguely remembered that she had mentioned Dr. Sarno to me before, but this time I finally took her comment to heart. As soon as I got home I promptly ordered Sarno's book from Amazon. There was not much to lose: his *Mindbody Prescription* [9] was $9.46 on Amazon, paperback edition, free shipment.

I had no idea how fateful that day was going to be.

Mindbody and TMS

The book arrived on February 16. By the end of next day, I got to the last page. My head was spinning. On one hand, the book promised a miracle. On the other hand, I knew darn well that miracles did not exist. On one hand, the book put the control over recovery from chronic pain squarely in the hands of a patient, which was so much better than dealing with the maze of the healthcare system. On the other hand, it left me with a full responsibility for my recovery. It made me feel equally liberated by putting power in my hands (no pun intended), and burdened with the work of healing, which, looking back, was much harder than I initially thought it would be.

I must refer the reader to Dr. Sarno's books for a complete explanation of his theory and detailed account of his successes over decades of practice. But here is my very brief interpretation of his book, which by no means replaces the original.

Dr. Sarno started as a physician in a very orthodox way, which was to accommodate or fix the structural defects in the patients' backs: bulging discs, deformed vertebrae, inflammation etc. He followed the official guidelines, prescribed physiotherapy, medications, and whatever else he was taught to do.

However, as an attentive and thoughtful observer, he soon noticed that quite a few people continued to have recurring pain problems, after many of the non-invasive treatments or even invasive surgeries that were supposed to "fix" the problems. Some people had multiple surgeries performed on their spines, to no effect. Or, to put it more accurately, to no healing effect. There were certainly effects on their wallets due to the high cost of treatments, and also the side effects caused by surgeries and medications, but not much in terms of disappearing pain.

Especially puzzling were cases where pain seemed to be associated with a certain time of the day or a season, or certain life situations but not the others. He also noticed that there were some mind-bending studies done on back pain. He cited one in which x-rays of the patients' backs with pain and without pain were done and it showed that the patients without pain complaints were nearly as likely as patients with pain complaints to have deformities in their spines. There was no correlation between structural "issues" with the spines and actual pain. He also was wondering how, in a very comfortable and physically undemanding modern life, our society ended up with the epidemic of back pain that got worse over the last decades, especially as fewer and fewer people had to do any physically challenging work.

At the time, Dr. Sarno also had a friend, a psychiatrist who practiced Freudian psychoanalysis, and they talked about their respective areas of expertise and possible impacts of repressed emotions. It was thanks to the psychoanalyst friend that one day, Dr. Sarno was having another bout of migraine and decided to think about repressed anger as a cause of his migraine. He sat down and thought for a while – and, to his total surprise, his migraine went away. He repeated his trick a few times – and it worked again and again. That got Dr. Sarno thinking about the nature of the pain and its possible roots in the emotional stresses of life.

Sarno coined the term TMS (Tension Myositis Syndrome) to describe the phenomenon of emotion-induced pain. His followers now spell out acronym TMS as The Mindbody Syndrome.

Eventually, Dr. Sarno developed a radical and controversial method that earned him scorn from colleagues and admiration of the patients, including celebrities like radio host Howard Stern and U.S. Senator Tom Harkin. The evidence of his success was a website titled "Thank you, Dr. Sarno," where dozens of stories of recovery were posted.

Thousands of patients were healed by listening to a two-hour lecture given by Dr. Sarno in a group setting, followed by a Q&A session. There were only two conditions that Dr. Sarno required from the patients to qualify for his treatment:

1. Dr. Sarno had to examine them and determine that there was no actual structural damage like broken bones or tumors in their spines; bulging discs counted as a normal wear and tear that our spines were designed to handle.
2. They had to accept that their pain had a psychological origin of some kind and that nothing was wrong structurally with their backs.

Half of his patients decided that the proposed approach was not credible and left, but another half stayed. Of those, about 80% recovered in a few weeks following the lecture. The remaining 20% were referred to a hand-picked group of psychologists that Sarno worked with. Of those, most also recovered.

He also noticed that these patients often possessed A-type personalities and were successful entrepreneurs or professionals – people who otherwise thrived in the high-pressure American life. They also often had histories of childhood abuse or emotional traumas.

Sarno described a story of a woman who suffered for years from crippling severe back pain, until one day a very painful memory of the sexual abuse by a family member floated to the surface of her consciousness. The memory was so painful that her mind had chosen to push it aside and keep it there for years. Upon recollection of this long-forgotten trauma, she went into the state of severe rage, cried and wept for several days, but when she emerged from her rage, her back pain disappeared and never returned.

Another proof of his theory was the first book that he published. He started receiving letters from those who read his book and saw their chronic pain disappear - from simply knowing and understanding the cause of their pain.

At the end of the book, Sarno listed about a dozen other conditions that he thought could also be caused by TMS. Migraines, Irritable Bowel Syndrome (IBS), ulcers, colitis, allergies, etc. may all be a result of repressed emotions.

Both CTS and CRPS/RDS were listed, although the section on CRPS/RDS had only one case of a successful recovery, and the patient's condition did not even vaguely resemble mine. But as I started putting together all the prior chronic conditions that bothered me throughout my life, a picture consistent with Dr. Sarno's theory started shaping up. Reynaud's, migraines, lower and upper back pain came and went, but in my adult life I almost always had one of the TMS conditions from Dr. Sarno's list. I also possess what Dr. Sarno's describes as a TMS personality: overachiever, often hard on myself, people-pleaser. If it wasn't a bingo, it did look like a good match.

While I was willing to accept that my problems had their roots repressed emotions, I was not quite sure about how to start on this path, nor had I any confidence that I would be among those lucky ones who succeed.

Still, it was hope versus despair, 80% chance of recovery versus only 20%, full control of my destiny versus reliance on unpredictable surgeries, medications, insurance companies. I had little to lose and a lot to gain. Even if it was a placebo, a placebo that I believed in, a placebo that would bring a recovery, it was better than the treatments that I did not believe in. I decided to go for it.

Forums

A quick step back from my main timeline – but nevertheless important. As I was tirelessly and desperately googling my way through the convoluted world of the online CRPS knowledge base, I came across forums. At first, I felt relief that I had found a community.

The sense of isolation created by my mysterious and crippling condition is hard to describe. You feel alone in your struggle. Doctors may be sympathetic, but you get to see them for 20 minutes, which are mostly taken by their usual rituals: they ask you what brought you into the office, you tell them about your symptoms, then quick examinations and maybe a minute or two of them explaining to you what you may already know. Then they write a prescription or not – and then they must move onto the next patient, leaving you alone up against your illness.

And it was not just illness. I was embarrassed to admit to my boss that I could not drive on business assignments, that I could not write notes, that I could not open certain doors in the office building. Looking back, I understand that all those embarrassments were nonsensical creations of my mind, caused by exhaustion from pain, insomnia, and fear. Many people live with much worse impairments and come to terms with the blows their fate deals them. But this is how I felt. I was stressing over going to HR and asking for special accommodations. I was scared and embarrassed of being incapacitated and didn't really have anybody to talk about it.

Forums were a different story. We all were in the same boat. There were newcomers like me, asking questions. There were veterans who had spent years in their misery, and they were glad to share their knowledge with the newcomers. There was plenty of information to go around, but the CRPS forum turned out to be a very depressing place. As I continued searching for keywords "full recovery," "partial recovery," or "remission" – I kept coming up almost emptyhanded.

It did look like the official stats on CRPS were not lying: Reports of recovery were an exception, not a rule. Most people had been on the forum for a long time, and the newcomers arrived at a steady pace. The air of resignation to inevitability of pain was thick. Suffering and misery seeped out of nearly every word posted on that forum. I vividly remember one thread, where people were sharing photos of their limbs devastated by CRPS. Swollen beyond recognition, hands, arms, feet, and legs were red, purple, and even blackish.

One man posted a photo of his legs engulfed in CRPS all the way up above the knees. He was begging his doctors to amputate his leg and was hoping to succeed. To suffer so much from pain that amputation seemed a success – what an awful way to live a life! It has been more than three years ago, but I still remember my shock and horror upon seeing those images – as if it was yesterday.

Most ambitions of the forum members did not go beyond preventing CRPS from spreading. Some patients were using ketamine, a drug that was not covered by insurance companies, for the chronic pain. Ketamine shots are very expensive. Each treatment can cost thousands of dollars, while the effect lasts only a few months. Many people who had been ill for a long time were on disability and could not afford ketamine.

However, I found occasional stories of some miraculous recoveries through brain stimulation. I also found videos on YouTube, advertising dental implants from a couple of medical offices, and reports of miraculous but undisclosed techniques employed by a couple of doctors in Europe.

But then I came across a series of posts by a woman who was able to recover from a severe case of CRPS. In addition to pain and hypersensitivity in her arms, she had a severe dystonia. Her arm was firmly bent in a bizarre position and was pushing against her head, forcing her head to tilt. She could not wear normal clothes and spent her days trying to find poses in which she could be more comfortable.

Judging by her story, she was incredibly brave and industrious. She found a doctor in Atlanta, who treated patients with brain stimulation. For out-of-town patients, he would send them home with a device that they could purchase from him and the instructions to use it. The initial set of parameters on the device this woman received from his office did not result in any changes in her condition, so she started experimenting with the settings, until she found certain parameters at which her brain suddenly flipped the switch. Her arm relaxed and dropped, and pain disappeared. However, the symptoms soon returned, so she had to repeat the procedure, but less and less frequently. Eventually the stimulation was no longer needed and she was free from pain and dystonia.

She was very generous and kind to others on the forum, answering endless questions. Several people followed her path and went to see that doctor. However, despite their attempts to use a prescribed set of parameters on the device, and then a modified set of parameters, they did not get better. After a couple years of patiently consulting people on the forum, the woman stopped answering the questions and, probably, moved on with her normal life, leaving the house of horrors behind.

I took note of her story and checked out the website of the Atlanta doctor. I even talked to him. He was honest. He estimated chances of improvement at about two out of three and readily admitted that he could not explain why and how brain stimulation made the pain and spasms go away. But he knew that his method helped quite a few people and was willing to offer help to those who wanted to take their chances. I was too scared to try the device – what if it changed something in brain that I would not want to change? However, his story added credibility to Dr. Sarno's theory that the brain, not the compressed local nerves, was the cause of the problems in my hands.

There was, however, one thread on the CRPS forum that set my hopes very high. At the time I came across that thread, I already knew about Dr. Sarno. There was a woman, Ines, who recovered from CRPS by reading Sarno's book. I could not find any indication of how bad her condition was or how long it took to go away. She was rather brief and gave a single explanation of her method: She just kept reading the book until the pain went away. People on the forum were incredulous and kept asking, looking for a caveat or secret additional details. Her response was the same: I just kept reading. I don't remember how many times I re-read her posts. It must have been dozens. I was slowly building up my fragile hope that I may be able to recover by using Dr. Sarno's method.

I can see how somebody who struggled with CRPS for years would flat out refuse to accept the idea that one can recover from such a complex and threatening illness by reading a book. It would put in question the years of suffering, exorbitant costs of treatments, and the very foundation of the modern clinical medicine. Many people could not accept it. Maybe because I was only few months into my CRPS misery, my mind was not conditioned enough to accept CRPS as inevitability. I knew I had to try.

I stopped reading the rest of the posts on that forum – I didn't want the talk about ketamine injections or physical therapy or painkillers to distract from the path I had chosen.

Nothing Is Wrong With My Body – But How Do I Know?

Dr. Sarno always started treatment of his patients by making sure that they did not have an actual structural problem. The key was that his definition of structural problem was different from the conventional view, which defined minor abnormalities as a potential root cause of pain.

But this is where my problem was: I didn't have Dr. Sarno around to check me out. I was more than willing to travel to New York to see him, but he had already retired.

So far, every doctor that I had seen told me that nerves in my hands showed substantial degradation, which was proven by the nerve conduction study. Shiny red skin, swelling and clenched fingers were other evidence of structural problems with my body.

To make matters worse, I didn't have ANY doctor who would even agree with me that I had CRPS. I had plenty of doctors who were quite certain that I had carpal tunnel syndrome (CTS), which was also listed in Sarno's book as a TMS condition, but this is where my mind was uncompromising. Somehow, I could not get my mind off the idea that my CRPS diagnosis had to be confirmed.

So, I decided to check back in with the neurologist, Dr. W. I walked into the Dr. W's office with the copy of *Mindbody Prescription* in my hand. I didn't expect much from my appointment, but Dr. W. really came through for me. He was friendly and willing to listen. After I explained that I wanted my diagnosis to be set straight and told him about the Budapest Criteria, he turned to his computer, did some Google searches, and quickly conceded that I met all the conditions for CRPS. But, he added, you still have symptoms of CTS.

The conversation wasn't as smooth when it came to the idea of psychosomatically induced neurological conditions. While Dr. W. agreed that stress could trigger muscle tensions and spasms, he nevertheless was not willing to consider the repressed emotions as a key factor in such profoundly physical symptoms like swelling, changes in skin color or dystonia, let alone the well- documented degradation in the ability of my nerves to conduct electrical signals. Even more

69

so, he was not willing to dismiss the diagnose of CTS (carpal tunnel syndrome).

I realized that he helped me the best he could – so I thanked him and left his office for good.

Meanwhile, the time came for me to start the program at the pain management clinic at The Clinic. I was hoping to find some support for Sarno's ideas among the specialists there. I was in for a disappointment.

It Is All in My Head

I am now almost ready to get to the next chapter, which focuses on my path to recovery. But before I move on, I feel it is necessary to share my last couple stories about the mainstream pain medicine.

One of the key recommendations from Dr. Sarno was to immediately discontinue any treatments that aim at fixing structural issues. That was easy.

By then, I had stopped seeing the acupuncturist. I came to the conclusion that K. did the best he could: He reduced my neuropathic pain and improved my sleep - somewhat. It was clear to me that he could not cure my dystonia. Something else was there at play that he could not fix. I sent him a polite and cordial thank-you note and cancelled all upcoming appointments.

The only treatment I was still pursuing was physical therapy with Leigh. Thirty-minute appointments with Leigh were happening less and less frequently. She started telling me that she had taught me everything she could. But her sessions were providing me with structure and simply a little bit of warmth and compassion, which I so much needed at the time.

One day, I brought Sarno's book to my appointment. But when I excitedly started telling Leigh about my newfound knowledge, her reaction was rather off-putting. She said, "Don't tell anybody that your pain is psychologically induced. They would think that it is all in your head." At that time, I didn't find the right words. I know now what I should have told her: "If I get to choose between a something-in-my-head that I can control and make go away and a something-in-my-body that nobody can make go away, I would rather have that something-in-my-head."

But back then, I really did not know what to say. Instead, I asked her whether any of her prior patients recovered from CRPS. Her answer was "They got better, but they did not recover." There was no cruelty in her words, just an honest acknowledgement that she really didn't know what else she could do for me. I do not recall whether I saw her again after that conversation.

I feel no disappointment toward Leigh, instead, I remember her with sincere gratitude. She was an honest professional and spoke the truth she knew. Her entire training and years of practice taught her a completely opposite approach. She was not prepared to treat that "something" that was in her patient's head.

Thank you, Dr. L

Pain management clinics are a relatively recent development in our society. They mushroomed in the 1970s and 1980s, when some researchers concluded that pain by itself was a medical condition, and so patients should be treated for chronic pain by the painkillers. No wonder that often physicians in charge of pain management clinics are anesthesiologists. You must agree, anesthesiologists are powerful. The stuff the anesthesiologist administered into my bloodstream for my appendectomy felt so heavenly - it still makes me nostalgic 10 years later. With never-ending pain, I felt temptation to just fill Dr. B's prescription and forget about pain and all my life problems along with it – but I knew about the potential consequences of addiction very well and was scared to start on the slippery path.

The Clinic's pain management clinic I was referred to was not an exception. The director was anesthesiologist, Dr. L. He was a young man, very energetic and very proud of his recent training at the Stanford Pain Clinic, to which he referred frequently throughout our first appointment.

In addition to Dr. L, the clinic had three psychologists who all happened to know about Sarno. One of them had studied psychoanalysis, and the idea of repressed emotions was well familiar to her. She was interested in working with me, but we never got past, among other things, her habit of listening to me for couple minutes and then repeating what I just said back to me and asking, "So, what do you think?" Well, I just spent two minutes telling you what I think – why are you asking me back? So, I stopped seeing her and decided to just stick with the class on pain management, which I found very helpful.

The class was taught by another psychologist and focused mostly on how to cope with pain. Her guided meditation sessions at the end of the class were short (five minutes) but very good. She seemed to have an endless supply of hugs, warm heartfelt advice, and encouragement for her students who were all long suffering from chronic pain.

But I soon realized that, while learning how to cope with pain was very helpful as an interim tactical step, it did not help me to achieve my ultimate goal: to get rid of both pain and dystonia.

Looking back, I know that I made the right decision. The entire concept of pain management assumes that chronic pain stays with the patient till death do them part. Being a successful business model for those providers who view medicine as business, it is not very helpful to the patients who are handed a life sentence of misery. I have no doubt that within the system of pain management clinics there are many honest professionals who are trying, sincerely and with compassion, to support the victims of chronic pain throughout their life of misfortune. But the main premise remains the same: You may reduce your pain with painkillers or increase your tolerance to pain with mental exercise, but the pain will never go away.

So, I moved on. But not until I was summoned to appear again in front of Dr. L. Dr. L clearly was eager to convince me to try some painkillers. He pulled out an iPad and started showing me diagrams and anatomical charts explaining in detail the mechanism of chronic pain. After a while, I asked him if the medications he wanted me to try would uncurl my curled fingers, but he was not sure. He was sure, however, that pain could be greatly reduced with the medication.

When I mentioned Dr. Sarno, Dr. L became a bit annoyed and told me that he had an issue with Dr. Sarno. Dr. Sarno, in his opinion, was too radical. While the concept of physical pain being caused by a signal from the brain was acceptable to Dr. L, the idea that a signal of physical pain could be sent by the brain in response to emotional pain sounded too radical to him.

I thought to myself that with full respect for his years of training, I could certainly accept his logic, however the question remained: Why then there is a website "Thank you, Dr. Sarno!" but no website "Thank you, Dr. L!"?

Being a polite person, I didn't say that out loud. Looking back now, I wish I had. Not to make my point, but hopefully to wake Dr. L up to the idea that a mainstream point of view de jour is not always right. Remember when lobotomy was the mainstream direction of neurological clinical practice?

Thinking Psychologically

As I am writing these chapters, I re-read *Mindbody Prescription*. While reading this book now as an "outsider" to my past pain, I wonder why it took me so long to be convinced. Dr. Sarno is very concise, clear, and persuasive in explaining his theory. He operates with statistical data he has collected in decades of practice. Why was it so hard for me to become convinced? From my experience interacting with dozens of people who faced the same problem, I came to understand why it is so hard to think psychologically.

Many TMS recovery stories start with how TMS sufferers first refused to read Sarno's book or even threw it away in anger because they refused to believe that their pain was "in their heads."

I observed how newcomers to TMS ask the same very basic question, time and over again, phrased differently under different angles and directed at different people, but the nature of the question is the same: Can it really be that my back (neck, foot, head – or insert your own favorite here) hurts because of the emotions? Not as frequently, but for a much longer time, people stumble through a harder question: Can it really be that the spasm in my back (leg, arm, hand –

or insert your favorite here) is happening because of the emotions?

And then there are those who struggle even more to believe that swelling, changes in the skin color and texture, rash, and many other very physical manifestations can be attributed to emotions. I know - because I was one of them. All those tangible, visible changes in your body are much harder to accept as a product of your mind than an invisible pain. When everything in your body seems to rebel against you, when pain, swelling, spasms, rash, bizarre, extremely painful red blotches on your skin, and what appears to be a paralysis of your limbs attack you from all sides, you are even less likely to become convinced. It is hard to believe that this total surrender of the body to a pathology can be caused by emotions. Ironically, the only logical explanation seems to be that it must be caused by the overstressed nervous system and nothing else.

We are conditioned by mainstream medicine that all physical symptoms should be treated by the doctors as abnormalities of the body. We are also conditioned to believe that each part of our body must have its own specialist. The unfortunate truth of our healthcare system is that the only doctor who is expected to oversee the entire patient - a general practitioner - is so tied up by insurance guidelines, 20-minute appointments, an endless stream of patients, that he/she is often reduced to being a dispatcher who refers patients out to the specialists, who, in turn, focus on their respective body parts. A podiatrist does not look above the ankle, a hand specialist is not allowed to think beyond the wrist, and a dermatologist is only prescribing ointments and creams to reduce itching or pain of the skin.

Our healthcare system is designed to look at the individual trees but not at the entire forest of a human being. Note, that none of those hand, foot, eye specialists are expected or even trained to consider psychological factors as both a cause of a disease and as a solution to it. In this situation, it is left to the patient herself to connect the dots into a big picture of a whole, that single mindbody in which everything is connected.

But this is what I understand now. Looking back, I can see how my mind, inflamed by severe pain, exhausted by years of persistent insomnia and recent months of even more extreme insomnia, weakened by the fear of inevitable progression of my symptoms to my other limbs, simply refused to accept a very logical conclusion.

Even though on an intellectual level I was able to quickly grasp Dr. Sarno's logic, it took me about a year of a long and winding path through doubt and hesitation, through frustration and despair, to get to the point. Yes, it took me a year to develop a firm, unshakeable belief that my illness was a result of my habitual subconscious suppression of emotions, which was hurting my already overstressed nervous system even more.

It was only then that I was able to feel confident that my recovery was inevitable. It was only then that I finally overcame the fear that was rooted deeply inside me on a subconscious level. And it was only then that I finally started to heal steadily.

By that time, guided by Dr. Sarno, I was able to picture together many manifestations of TMS that persisted throughout my life: bizarre sudden shortness of breath and spasms in my diaphragm that started in my pre-teens and then stopped completely after about 40 years; very painful shins that prevented me from exercising when I was a teenager; severe migraines that repeated three - four times per month and lasted one - three days each since I was 16 until I was in my 50s; lower back pain that hit me suddenly when I was in my early 40s; insomnia that started when I was in college and gradually became worse, leading to narcoleptic episodes, one of which nearly killed me on the road; two bad outbreaks of rosacea, one after a difficult pregnancy and childbirth, another after my mother was killed in a hit-and-run accident by a heavily drugged teenager; and then, the grand finale – neuropathic pain combined with Reynaud Syndrome and dystonia that almost disabled me completely. I was able to put each of the onsets on a timeline and match them fairly accurately to the traumatic events in my life.

But that was much later. Back in February of 2016, I was just starting on that path, scared, confused, and hesitant.

Throwing Away Crutches

One of the first recommendations from Sarno was to throw away crutches: Stop using any props or special accommodations for the painful conditions and resume normal physical activities.

By then, I had surrounded myself with props and limitations: gloves to keep my hands warm, grip gloves for the door handles and for the steering wheel, special keyboard at work, no driving on the freeways etc.

I had been sleeping on the couch for a couple of months by then. It was easier for me to sit upright, with both arms resting in a vertical position, preferably hanging down. It somehow kept my neuropathic pain at lower levels. I bought a large memory foam pillow to prop myself up against. This contraption, along with K.'s pills, allowed me a couple of stretches of two - three hours of shallow sleep at night – on a good day. But how do I possibly give up my pillow and my upright sleeping position if I can barely get any sleep even with these props? After a short hesitation, I decided to make a leap of faith.

To my complete surprise, after I relocated back to my bed, my sleep didn't get worse. I still felt neuropathic pain, but somehow, as I started believing that maybe nothing was wrong with me structurally, it was easier for me to cope with the pain.

Once I discovered that my first crutch was so easy to dispose of, I tried to ditch the rest of them: grip gloves, forget-everything-you-like diet, Topricin, no driving on freeways, Aleve and Motrin. But that turned out to be much harder. Dystonia and pain were hitting me right back.

Forum of Hope

Of course, upon discovery of Dr. Sarno and TMS, I immediately started my Internet searches, now on TMS. I discovered that there was a lot of information on TMS out there, but mainstream medical sites did not talk about it.

As we all know, the Internet is full of information, both credible and not so credible. When it comes to this area of medicine, it is very easy to fall into the traps set up by the sellers of cure-everything pills, expensive recovery programs, etc. I was worried about it. Nevertheless, I found an online forum that seemed to be relatively well insulated from miracle pills and miraculous surgeries. No surprise, it was set up and run by the practitioners who followed Dr. Sarno's method, but also by former, now-recovered patients, mostly volunteers. Interesting that many of the practitioners affiliated with the TMS website had themselves recovered from chronic pain using Dr. Sarno's method and some of them were even his former patients or students.

This is what made that forum stand out: the hope that permeated the air. Of course, there were plenty of people in despair. There were those who could not succeed despite years of trying, but there were many more who had recovered. Those who recovered were helping those who were trying to recover. The most striking section of the website is called "Thank you, Dr. Sarno." I was told that it was a digital reincarnation of the binder full of letters of gratitude from Dr. Sarno's former patients that his staff kept in his office. The letters were so sincere and full of details that I started believing that Dr. Sarno was the real deal.

The amount of information on the forum was overwhelming. It was there that I learned about many other physicians, those who completely left the officially approved pain practice and those who managed to live in both worlds. One of them was Dr. Claire Weekes, a general practitioner from Australia who helped me tremendously to find my way, despite no longer being with us since the 1990s. Luckily for me, she left behind audio recordings, which I listened to almost every day for many months.

For about a year, I was on the forum for hours every day, first asking questions, but later mostly answering. As I started seeing improvement in my condition, I started helping other people to get through initial fog and uncertainty. I sometimes scan the most desperate posts that have not received a response for a day or two, just to give people a word of encouragement – like others did it for me. I still answer questions, and other members of the community sometimes send people my way if their questions pertain to CRPS or dystonia.

TMS Practitioners

TMS forum is a part of an umbrella web site, TMSWiki.org. For a chronic pain sufferer who just recently learned about TMS, TMSWiki can be overwhelming, as it is packed with information and resources.

You can find a list of TMS practitioners of various specialties, from physicians to psychologists. Some of the physicians who practice TMS-oriented medicine converted to the TMS approach after they became Dr. Sarno's success stories as patients. Some were patients of those who were helped by Dr. Sarno. They truly practice the "do unto others..." principle.

The site was created and is maintained by PPD/TMS Network, association of practitioners who treat TMS or, using a more descriptive term, psychophysiologic disorders (PPD). Alan Gordon, probably the most prolific contributor to the site, generously publishes healing frameworks and answers questions from the members of the forum. Use of the site is free, which makes it accessible even for people who cannot afford to pay for the consultations.

As I dove into the sea of information on the site, I learned a lot, but it did not ease my doubts about the validity of Dr. Sarno's method for CRPS and about my own abilities to succeed. Leigh's sobering assessment of my prospects with CRPS ("they got better, but they did not recover") stuck in my head. Most importantly, I still could not buy into the idea that my irreparably damaged nerves could recover. Anxious and fearful, I decided to check with a TMS-practicing physician.

Go figure, my obsessive mind needed a neurologist to counter the verdict given me by Dr. W and the rest of the official medicine. Surprisingly, even that option was available through the magic of TMSWiki and Internet. Dr. Roger Geitzen was born into a family of physicians and was destined to follow the family trade. However, his very conventional medical training did not dissuade his interest in alternative medicine. He studied with Dr. Andrew Weil, a renowned Harvard-trained physician and author, whose book *Spontaneous Recovery* benefited me greatly. He also studied with Dr. Schubiner, a student of Dr. Sarno.

I reached out to Dr. Geitzen. He agreed to look at my records and talk to me on Skype. My full set of The Clinic's records emailed to him ahead of time, I got on Skype. As I described my experiences in the maze of official healthcare, I felt by his response that he completely understood my disappointments. He reviewed my records and agreed with me that my symptoms had nothing to do with structural issues. In his opinion, I had TMS.

But then there was something else he had to tell me. In his neurology practice, he saw one patient with severe CRPS. One of her hands was impacted in the same way as mine. She endured multiple treatments and surgeries, but her condition only got worse. She ended up giving up on her impacted hand and relied on the healthy one. Despite this, Roger encouraged me to give Sarno's approach a shot. In a way, I had no other options but to go forward. I didn't have a healthy hand to rely on. Both of my hands were affected and were getting worse.

With Roger's encouragement and after giving up on the The Clinic's pain psychologists, I started looking for a TMS psychologist. TMS Wiki had a lot of material published by Alan Gordon, director of the LA Pain Psychology Center. I reached out to Alan, explained my symptoms – and the next day I got a call from Amber Murphy, a therapist at the Center who herself recovered from CRPS. Amber was a godsend. We had about 10 sessions over Skype. Amber was focused on just one goal: free me up from my fear. Week after week, she pounded one simple idea into my brain, from different angles and approaches: Don't be afraid.

I did something very important, following both Amber's advice and Alan's recovery plan on the TMS Wiki. I wrote a good-bye letter to my fear, which somehow increased my confidence in my future success. Generous with her time, always positive and inspirational, Amber succeeded. By the time we ended our sessions, I started feeling a little bit better.

Looking back, I cannot stop wondering why it took me so long to accept that I was terrified and paralyzed by my fears and that the fears were the cause of my CRPS. But I understand that I was not in a very rational state of mind during those days.

After 10 sessions, I realized that the benefits of talking to Amber on a weekly basis were outweighed by the frustrations over my unreliable Internet connection. We stopped formal sessions, but Amber and I stayed in touch for a couple of years after. She sent me links to the useful Internet sites, I reported my progress. Her enthusiastic response and unwavering faith in my ability to recover gave me a huge boost of self-esteem and determination. I am forever grateful to Amber.

But I realize that I have now arrived onto the next chapter, *Healing and Recovery.*

Chapter 5. Healing and Recovery
The Toolbox
In Chapter 5, I am going to describe the practitioners who I worked with and the tools that I used to recover, one per section. That does not mean that I used them one by one in a linear fashion. None of them individually was a magic bullet that worked instantaneously with a lasting impact. They all came together and often were used concurrently, but I was discovering and putting them to use rather one by one.

I cannot tell with certainty how each one of those practices contributed to my recovery. I did not have the luxury to set my experiments in a fully controlled way like in a clinical trial – I was fighting for my survival.

Sometimes, I did not see any results for weeks, but slowly things started improving. Once again, I cannot say with certainty which one of the methods worked, and to which degree. I do not have a hard proof that any one of them contributed to my success as an actual therapy and not as a placebo. But the placebo effect is well-known to the scientific community as a powerful tool – and if I recovered thanks to the placebo effect, I would take it over surgeries and opioids any time.

Some of the things I tried did not feel like a viable option after a while, but it very well could be that they would work for somebody else. Some of the things I have tried resulted in short-term improvements in my conditions and then my hands curled back again. However, whenever I witnessed my hands uncurled even for an hour, I knew that I was slowly helping my brain to unlearn the bizarre pattern it was stuck in.

I can only hope that maybe some researchers would be interested in working with people like me who overcame CRPS and dystonia and come up with some statistically proven methodologies.

Meanwhile, the readers should do what I have done: Try anything that seems reasonable and safe, keep doing everything that seems to work, be creative, flexible and chart your own path.

And remember, your healing path must start with realization and deep understanding of what led you to becoming sick. It took me many months to come to a full understanding of what happened to me and why. You too should not rush to the conclusions.

Cure vs. Healing

I heard this notion before: When you have an incurable disease, you cannot be cured, but you may be able to heal. It didn't mean much to me until, by stumbling and wandering on the healing path, I myself figured out what healing meant – at least what it meant to me.

My friend and teacher Kathleen told me one day, "You cannot take the key to your health and turn it over to a doctor, you have to be an active participant." As I learned, healing meant that I had to take an ultimate responsibility for my recovery. That did not mean that it was a sudden do-it-yourself miracle. No doubts, I relied on several healthcare professionals to help me out. But I knew that without my actively re-wiring my brain, my perceptions, my attitudes, and daily routines success would have not been possible.

Numerous studies showed that patients with a positive attitude tend to recover faster and more frequently even from very serious illnesses. There have been studies comparing religious and non-religious cancer patients and their recovery patterns. Good news for the believers: Religious patients showed better results than non-religious ones.

Not being a psychologist or a physician, I am attempting to explain the difference between cure and healing from my layman's point of view.

Picture a "bucket" of resources that your body needs to survive and thrive. Imagine that if there is a hole through which your resources are being depleted, the outflow would grow as you accumulate destructive pressures on your body along your life path. If you don't learn how to properly react to the pressures and prevent the hole from growing bigger, sooner or later you will lose the ability to replenish your "bucket."

Cure usually means that you physically "plug" the hole or increase the inflow of resources by getting surgery or taking medication. But an externally applied plug may not always stop the hole from re-opening again, which would require taking medication forever or repeat surgeries.

Healing means that you figure out how to absorb and dispose of negative effects of life pressures in a way that does not increase the drain on your resources. Healing means that you utilize the internal resources of your body and mind to become more resilient.

Everything in our body is connected, and the nervous system, being involved in every psychological and physiological process in our mind and body, can act either as a helper or as an enemy. It will mobilize and redirect your resources to where they are needed, or, if your internal resources are insufficient to overcome the stress, it will start diverting resources from other parts of the body to the one that is in crisis. By the same token, if we are worrying and stressing out when we are sick, we are putting additional undue pressure on the nervous system and re-directing our resources to unproductive activities, which worrying often is.

Robert Sapolsky, a neuroendocrinology professor at Stanford University, explains the mechanism of such mobilization in his book *Why Zebras Don't Get Ulcers*. Luckily, I read his book years before I got sick, and my knowledge came in very handy. It gave me a frame of reference and a compelling explanation of why I got sick. Sapolsky describes how, at times of great danger, the body of an animal switches to the "fight or flight" mode. All the bodily functions that can be suspended while the animal fights the attacker or flees - such as digestion - automatically shut down, giving all the resources to the legs and arms, to fight back or to run as fast as possible.

That explains why at times of great stress and danger people throw up, wet or soil their pants: Our body prepares us, much like it did for our ancestors, to dump whatever is in our bowels or our stomach. Why? To get rid of the stuff that may slow us down on the run or may make it harder to fight the attacking tiger. And here is the difference between humans and zebras. Zebras live in the moment. Once the tiger is gone, zebra goes back to its peaceful life, and forgets the stress. But humans nowadays rarely face a real tiger. Today a "tiger" is a loss of a job, bankruptcy, burnout at work, or abusive partner. Or verbal abuse by the boss, who herself may be suffering from her own personal "tigers" and takes it out on you, just because you are an easy target. In this situation, a danger is prolonged and mostly psychological.

We cannot run or fight back. We just continue to endure. In addition, our brains are more advanced than the ones of zebras, which means that it is harder for us to forget about this psychological danger. Nevertheless, biologically we are identical to the humans of 50,000 years ago, who never had to face bankruptcy or divorce, or foreclosure that hangs over your head every day.

Sapolsky's book title makes it clear that ulcers and possibly some other modern illnesses are the result of stresses that people in our modern society cannot cope with. It is thanks to the paradigm of fight or flight described in Sapolsky's book that I eventually made a connection between the involuntarily contraction of my tendons and daily stresses of my life. Once the stress exceeded a certain threshold, my body began preparing to fight the tiger, unbeknownst to my mind. My muscles tightened up and my sleep became extremely disturbed. At some point, some pain-related circuits activated in my brain and led to the development of the complex regional pain syndrome.

In his *Mindbody Prescription*, Dr. Sarno lists dozens of major stressors in life that may lead to the development of chronic pain, in the descending order of impact. Of the stressors from Sarno's list, I had experienced several most destructive ones in several years preceding my illness.

Each one of them made a dent on my nervous system and opened a drainage hole in the resource pool of my body. The damage accumulated to the point where cure, even if it existed, would have not helped, as my body lost the ability to pick up a recovery pace on its own. Hence, every treatment I started in my first few months was destined to fail as my body could no longer mobilize its healing abilities. My body was stuck, clenching my fingers, hopelessly trying to fight the non-existent tiger. Day or night, my brain was alert, worried, and stressed out.

There was no way out of my illness other than re-training my brain out of the worries, obsessions, and pain. Recognition of it started my healing process.

Insomnia

I started sleeping poorly when I was in college. By my 30s, I had chronic, persistent insomnia. I woke up almost every night between 2:45 a.m. and 3:15 a.m., with a precision of the atomic clock. Occasionally, I was able to go back to sleep around 5 a.m., only for the alarm clock to ring at 6 a.m. More often though, I would turn and toss in bed until 6 a.m. without sleep, overwhelmed by the worries of my life, by the family troubles, by the instability at work, by the fears of how I would make it to the next paycheck or through the next month, or the next year. To make matters worse, even those few hours of sleep between 10 p.m. and 3 a.m. would not make me feel rested. My sleep was shallow. I woke up every hour or so. I dreaded going to bed as much as I dreaded getting up in the morning.

I also noticed that I was no longer having dreams. Not that I was missing strange and often disturbing visions that visited me at night when I was young, but I knew that dreams were linked to the REM phase of sleep, which carried a restorative function. I knew that something was amiss.

I tried sleeping pills, and I tried behavioral therapy, but Ambien and CBT did not work at all. I was told that I had sleep apnea and was offered a CPAP device, but noise from the pump would not let me go to sleep, so I declined.

At some point, I had an epiphany. I realized that when I woke up at 3 a.m., I was usually in the state of fear, and so my insomnia was a result of anxiety. I talked to the CBT therapist and was eventually given a prescription for Xanax. Xanax became a miracle drug for me. For about seven years, the lowest dosage of Xanax taken in the middle of the night made me go back to sleep after 20-30 minutes. But eventually Xanax stopped working. Increase in dosage did not help. I started getting hangovers and headaches in the morning, so I stopped taking Xanax. Without Xanax, life became very difficult. I often spent my waking time in a twilight condition: too exhausted to fall asleep and not able to do anything productive.

Insomnia made driving a car very difficult. The irony of the situation was that driving in stop-and-go traffic made me fall asleep reliably and quickly, especially on the freeways. I learned to pull off the freeway at the first sign of sleepiness and take a quick, refreshing nap in my car on the side of the road.

But one day, after the onset of sleepiness, it took me about three endless minutes to make it to the next off-ramp in slow traffic. I was already in the safety of the ramp when my brain shut down for a few seconds. When I opened my eyes, the car was rolling downhill, through the green belt, between the trees and bushes toward the busy street. Then it jumped a good three feet down off the retaining wall, shook violently, but kept going across the lanes. I was able to stop it a foot away from the tall brick wall dividing the street. My new car was wrecked by the debris it hit along the way, but it didn't hit other cars, and I was unharmed physically. Still, I was terrified and scarred emotionally. I became afraid of driving. I no longer trusted my ability to drive safely, which, of course, increased my anxiety levels. The accident happened two years before I became sick. I became even more careful and cautious about my driving, and my insomnia kept getting worse.

Fast forward two years, to December of 2015. No wonder additional worries over becoming disabled sent my already-fragile sleep spinning out of control. The herbs prescribed by the acupuncturist helped me to sleep somewhat, but they never brought me deep refreshing sleep, that instant blissful descent into the soft embrace of darkness I had experienced as a child.

As I struggled with insomnia, I thought that losing the ability to sleep well was part of the inevitable aging process. To my total surprise, within a few weeks from reading Sarno's book, I noticed that my sleep started improving. This takes me to the next section, Mindfulness.

Mindfulness

There is entire school of thought in clinical psychology revolving around mindfulness. The concept of mindfulness (aka awareness) came from the Buddhist teachings. Being aware of yourself, your mind, your thoughts, and your behavior is an important aspect of Buddhism. Mindfulness, as it is taught in the West, is often stripped of any references to its Buddhist roots, to make it more acceptable to non-Buddhists. One of the most prominent advocates of mindfulness in the U.S. is Jon Kabat Zinn who established a program for stress reduction at the University of Massachusetts in 1979.

Dr. Sarno may have not been aware of the Buddhist teachings when he discovered that by acknowledging his emotional distress he could make his migraine go away. But his ideas correlate very well with the teachings of mindfulness.

When one becomes mindful of her surroundings and starts observing her own behavior, emotions and thoughts as if looking from the outside, without personal attachment or dwelling on her feelings, she may start noticing the change. She may notice that each time she consciously tells herself: "Yes, I am angry. Yes, I feel anger burning in my chest, in my arms, I am very upset, but I am going to concentrate on how my anger feels in my body and how the burning sensation slowly dissipates in my body." Surprisingly, this little exercise, once repeated enough times, can become a habitual meditative practice for your mind and your body and result in changes. As it did for me. Our brains are plastic. Even when we are old, we can still change.

I started observing my reactions to the stresses of the day and recognizing emotions underneath my reactions. And I started clearly naming them to myself: anger, fear, sadness, joy.

Not being a clinical psychologist or neuroscientist, I would not dare to explain the mechanics of it, but the more I was thinking about my emotions and looking for the unresolved anger, sadness, or fear, the less vivid were my anxiety attacks at 3 a.m., the more likely I was able to "feel through" my anxiety and go back to sleep. And the better I slept, the less likely I was going to wake up the following night because I was not as exhausted and worried during the day and because I obsessed less over the negative aspects of my life.

I started having dreams again. Sometimes they were vague and unmemorable, but often they had a plot, cast, and colors – a short movie of a kind, much like dreams I had in my childhood. The emotions during my sleep were vivid and physical. I felt them in my body, not just in my mind. I was no longer scared of bad dreams: I welcomed them as a necessary release of negative emotions, a housekeeping practice of my brain.

I now often slept for six - seven hours without waking up, and in the morning felt refreshed and full of energy. The more observant and mindful I became of my emotional state, the more I understood how my life was often guided by unjustifiable fear and anxiety.

Mindfulness requires frequent practice, preferably daily. And the way to become truly mindful, or, in Buddhist terms, enlightened, is to meditate.

Meditation

Meditation is an exercise in mindfulness.

Meditation, an essential component of ancient healing arts like Ayurveda or Chinese medicine, requires more discipline and commitment from the patient than taking herbs or lying on the table for an acupuncture session. So, in our Western world of instant gratification, meditation as a healing procedure is not likely to be recommended even by the most sophisticated practitioners of Chinese medicine.

For those skeptical of meditation as a healing practice, I recommend that you explore the website from the National Institute of Health [11].

If anyone told me three years ago that I would be able to sit still for an hour and a half "not doing anything" – I would not have believed them. As a matter of fact, I prided myself on being an energetic go-getter who needed to be on the move all the time. A long-time yoga practitioner, I could never succeed in savasana – a corpse pose, which is a form of meditation. Rarely could I stop going over my to-do list, or dwelling on an unpleasant conversation at work, or thinking about what to cook for dinner while in savasana.

Years ago, as I learned about meditation from a book on yoga, I tried a guided group meditation once, but could not last for more than five minutes. I found sitting still an unbearable and useless exercise. As it turned out, "not doing anything" was hard work and it had a purpose that I didn't understand at the time. So, I never meditated - until the threat of disability became so real that I was willing to try just about anything.

One day, I read on the CRPS forum that meditation helped someone to reduce pain symptoms. It was consistent with what I learned at the pain clinic, so I signed up for the meditation class. A one-day class consisted of about four, 45-minute meditations, with talks and breaks in between. It was hard, but I stuck through it.

After taking the meditation class, I started meditating daily in the evening. It was hard. My mind would start wandering, my anxiety would start rising about 10-15 minutes into it. To make matters worse, I was in pain from sitting still. As I was sitting, I experienced increase in pain not only in my hands, but also in my arms, legs, and feet. Since I lost flexibility in my joints to dystonia, I could not sit on the floor cross-legged anymore, so I had to use a chair, but the pain was still present.

I tried all kinds of meditation: guided, unguided, walking, sitting, with music or without music – until I finally found my groove.

I soon found out that a guided meditation did not work for me in any form. I was too easily distracted by the voice of the instructor, by the instructions he/she was giving me, but most of all, by the prescriptive nature of instructions. I could not focus on my breath, whether it was on the count of four, or two, or any given number. Instructions were amplifying my anxiety.

Body scan, one of the most popular forms of self-guided meditation, did not work for me either. A prescribed sequence in which I was supposed to focus on relaxing my toes, then feet, then ankles, then legs etc. - until I reached my face - was an annoyance. I would get lost in thoughts halfway along my body or forget whether I took care of my right side before switching to the left side and so on. I bought various audio guides on meditation and tried to follow recommendations on proper cross-legged sitting, on keeping my back straight, on counting the elephants instead of breaths – and was getting nowhere. Especially hard was sitting cross-legged, since my joints were painful and cemented by dystonia.

I finally decided to just sit on the couch, rest my arms on the pillows, close my eyes, and do nothing: no counting of breaths, no body scan, no imagining a beautiful trail in the woods or a place where I wanted to be as a child.

Surprisingly, the less effort I put into following the rules, the better results I was getting. I came to believe that people like me who tend to be obsessive perfectionists and over-achievers, are too uptight and tense to follow instructions. Any perceived deviation from instructions was generating extra anxiety, thus ruining the experience. So, the best way to start was to abandon any prescriptions and ease my way into the practice, which is what I did.

Sitting Meditation

Once I put my mind to it, in a few weeks I was able to meditate for an hour or more, effortlessly. What was truly amazing, a day or two after a long meditation session, my pain level was a little bit lower. So, on Saturday and Sunday, I would meditate for an hour or as long as I could handle, and by Monday I would feel better.

Eventually, I found a few things that helped me even more in my meditation practice.

I learned that after about 15 minutes into the practice, my anxiety level would start rising, to the point that I would feel compelled to get up and do something: eat, check my email, do dishes, put a jacket on – anything to break the unbearable rendezvous with myself. Sometimes I would feel a rise in emotions, more often sadness or a sense of shame over some prior experience or even something that I could not identify. The simple act of acknowledging my anxiety and my feelings and telling myself that it was OK to be anxious somehow took the edge off it, and after another ten minutes of wrestling with my anxiety I would be calm and at peace.

Unlike guided meditation, very quiet rhythmic music was not distracting but rather helpful. I, however, went through a couple dozen tunes on YouTube that did not resonate well with me. Judging by the likes they earned, they were good for many people, but not for me at that moment. I found several that I use to date. They are soothing and calming on some days but not on others, so I choose the one that works for my mood of the day.

Somatic meditation, which is focusing on the sensations in the body and channeling emotions into the sensations, became my practice. (More on channeling the emotions into sensations in the section *Frozen Emotions*.)

I recognized that at the times of stress my stomach and belly turn into a tight knot. As I sit down for the meditation, I start with focusing on two areas, one above and one below the navel. For those familiar with Eastern healing arts, I am referring to a solar chakra and a hara chakra (dan tien). After about 20 minutes, I start feeling relaxed in that area and a heat wave starts rising in my body. Past that point, I enter the healing phase of meditation – at least what it feels to me. I find it very important to meditate for at least 30-40 minutes. The longer your session, the better the results. The same rule applies to all other types of meditational activities, which I will cover later. Being unconcerned with the end time of the meditation is also very important, as it removes undue stress and eases your way into the meditative state.

Short session or long, not every time do I feel the desired effect of meditation. I simply learned not to get upset if it does not work well on a certain day. Being able to let go of disappointment with yourself is a virtue. When I let go of my preconceived idea of how my meditation must proceed or end, I learned that there are many ways to achieve desired outcomes. Sitting meditation is not the only option. There are other types of meditative activities, such as swimming, walking, running, or watching the ocean waves. They do not become a meditation unless you are undertaking them mindfully, i.e. paying attention to sensations in your body, letting the thoughts that race through your mind come and go, recognizing your emotions and thoughts as manifestations of a restless mind.

I always loved swimming, and a once-a-week swim became a godsend during my first year of recovery when I was still in severe pain. Swimming is very gentle on the muscles, and it helped me a lot by stretching them without stressing them out. I also made sure that I swam at least one kilometer at a time, eventually increasing my regimen to a mile, so I could achieve a meditative effect over the course of 40 minutes or longer.

More on another form of the active meditation that I use – in the section *Running Meditation*. One day, I wrote down what was going on in my mind during my weekly runs.

Running Meditation

One - two, one - two – I hear my feet stamping on the trail. One - two, one - two. Forty-five minutes once a week – that's all the time I can spare for now. One - two, one - two.

I don't really run, I jog. I run around the lake near my office. A paved trail winds around the lake, but in some places, there is a parallel dirt trail, which I prefer to the pavement. I had been working near the lake for eight years before I put this trail to good use during my lunch hour. Until then, I used to work through lunch every day. I made a point of carving out a couple lunch breaks per week for myself, one for a run, one for Qi gong or yoga.

I run counter clock-wise, with the lake to my left, city noise to my right. The trail is flat, which adds monotony to my run. Monotony is much welcome. It calms down my anxiety and releases tension.

I meet some runners on the way. Some of them I even recognize – we are regulars. Most runners who run in the same direction pass me and leave me behind. I am slow, they are fast. Normally a competitive person, I don't care. I don't run for speed. I run for endurance, but even more so, I run for meditation.

For the first 10-15 minutes of my run, the office events swirl in my brain. Meeting that I forgot to schedule, report that I didn't finish, the email that was interrupted in the middle because somebody wanted to talk to me. Shopping list for tonight, weekend plans, phone call to a friend. I let the thoughts come and go, I don't dwell on them. One - two, one - two, I keep running. I watch the ducks in the water on my left, I notice little kids playing on the grass to my right. I pass young moms pushing strollers and old ladies walking slowly in pairs. The thoughts come and go, my feet stamp the ground, I keep running. I watch the blue sky, reflections of the clouds on water, I feel the wind on my face.

One - two, one - two, I keep running. Around the one-mile mark - or 15 minutes into it - something changes in me. I feel anxiety rising, I start feeling sad, I want to stop. I want to turn around and go back to the office, to deal with the emergencies that must be happening while I am here running. I need to check my email. I need to check my voice messages. I must be missing something back there – I must go! But I keep running. I know that for the next few minutes I will experience sadness and even tears in my eyes – for no reason. I now know that it is normal. I may feel the increased sense of stress and nervousness. But it is the most welcome emotional release.

I noticed that I often felt the same during my yoga practice, at my aerobics classes, on my hikes, during sitting meditation. I often followed the urge and, unable to get through the surge of anxiety or depression, driven by desire to push the feelings away, to stop them, I walked out of the aerobics classes, stopped my yoga practice halfway through, turned around during the hikes. Thanks to my new understanding of the mind-body connection, I no longer stop. I feel my sadness, I let the wave roll over my body. One - two, one - two, I keep running. The loop around the lake is my friend. It leads me forward, it does not let me turn around.

By the mile-two mark, I am tired. I am now facing the midday sun. It is getting hot. The trail is usually crowded on this stretch. The road comes almost to the edge of the lake. It is not my favorite part of the run, but my rules are simple: Slowing down is OK, stopping or switching to a walk is not. I have to finish the entire 3.4-mile loop without ever running out of breath. My pace is measured. It is just enough for my mind to slow down, for racing thoughts to fade away, for emotions to wear out.

When I am about half a mile away from the end of my run, my mind clears, I gain energy, I start speeding up. The ducks on the lake salute me. Sun is no longer burning my face. The wind picks up and cools my face. I finish my run with more energy than I started with. I feel victorious. My stress level is down. I am back to the office, but it feels like a homerun. I get through the rest of the day with a smile.

I started running after I got sick. At one of the lowest points in my CRPS saga, I got an email at the office inviting employees to join the annual 5K run. Never a runner before, I started thinking about doing it. Mainly to prove to myself that I was still capable of an achievement, to lift my spirit.

So, I ran my first 5K and I loved it. It was meditative, but also it was an exercise that didn't involve my arms and hands. My legs were in severe pain for two days after, but I loved even the pain – it was a pain of victory. Subsequently, I ran several half-marathons, and each of them gave me a new understanding of myself, my mental strength, and my physical abilities.

Two people helped me make up my mind about getting into half-marathons, incidentally, both were named Steve. SteveO – Steve Ozanich, a well-known figure on the TMS forum, who pulled himself out of severe disability following Dr. Sarno's method and Other Steve – my dear friend and inspiration.

SteveO was bedridden by chronic pain for years. When he read Sarno's book, he started running, despite pain – and pain finally went away. SteveO wrote a book, which is a very popular TMS recovery guide, also referenced in the bibliography section at the end of my book.

Other Steve is an ultra-marathoner, who found running to be the best escape valve for his life pressures. It helped him pull through some very rough times. Other Steve explained the concept in the simplest terms: If you keep running, pain eventually goes away, by mile 33 or even by mile 10. You just need to have patience and keep running. For those who don't believe Other Steve, I can attest that he has, in fact, run 55K races, more than once.

This empiric observation from Other Steve correlates well with the TMS concepts. Once you detach your mind from your TMS pain, the brain stops generating the pain signals. It proved true in my case, too. When I started running, my feet and ankles were affected by pain and dystonia. The monotony of running somehow had a calming effect not only on my anxiety but also on my tendons and ligaments. By the time I was finishing my loop around the lake, the pain was usually gone. After first few months of weekly runs, dystonia in my feet was mostly gone.

I am still dismissing the idea of running a full marathon as insanity, but who knows what is going to happen in the future?

Yoga

I started practicing yoga almost 20 years ago, out of desperation, after I injured my back. Unable to walk, drive, sit, or lie in bed without severe pain, I was looking for a cure. My doctors offered me pain killers and muscle relaxants. Neither worked very well.

Somebody suggested yoga. I signed up for the class at my gym. For six months I went to the class without seeing any results. Still, I wanted to give it a fair trial, but mostly to get my money's worth out of my gym membership. After a while, I noticed a change, as my pain slowly started receding and I was able to gradually get back to my hiking, backpacking, aerobics, and other physical activities. I became a yogi. If I skipped yoga for a week – my body noticed. If I skipped it for a month – my body ached.

I have practiced yoga, with varying degree of devotion, since then. I learned that my always-tight muscles were less tight after a class. Never flexible before, I slowly developed the ability to do things that I could not do even in my teens: stretches, folds, a headstand, even a handstand on occasion. I enjoyed my newfound connection with my body. However, something else eluded me: I could not relax my mind. Even after a strenuous 90-minute yoga class, the stress of daily life was still rolling through my head as I was lying on the floor in savasana, the corpse pose.

When my hands and wrists became swollen and crippled, I could no longer do yoga. But even before that break in yoga practice, I noticed a change in my body.

My ankles, knees, and other joints were not normal. Practicing the same yoga asanas time and time again for years gives you a good gauge of your abilities at a given moment. You know how far you can push yourself in a twist or a bend. Every yogi knows that there are good days and bad days. With years of practice, it was easy for me to detect the change. My flexibility in the months preceding CRPS was not the same anymore. I could not get into the asanas that I used to do easily before. I thought it was just another sign of aging.

I did not put it all together until I was on my second year of recovery and felt comfortable enough to try yoga again. I certainly was completely out of shape after not practicing for almost two years. But in addition, my muscles were responding with violent cramps each time I tried to stretch them even a little bit. My very first downward facing dog (one of the very basic yoga poses) ended very quickly, not because of my still crippled hands, but because of the cramps in my ankles, in my feet, in my legs.

It was obvious to me that I had to start at a beginner's level and with the flavor of yoga that I never liked before because it was not athletic and challenging enough for me. It is called yin yoga, and it consists of slow, long stretches held for three - five minutes each. Forced into yin yoga by necessity, I soon got to liking it as I realized that it was another form of meditation. Gentle, low- intensity stretches in a quiet dimly lit studio eventually taught my muscles to relax. Cramps started slowly calming down. I learned how to respond to the cramps by closing my eyes, meditating, and trying to relax the muscles.

In the months that followed, I was able to gradually intensify my yoga practice. It is now almost back to where it was in the months preceding the onset of CRPS. I am hoping to advance beyond that level, but with the new wisdom that I gained from practicing mindfulness and self-awareness.

Nowadays, yoga to me is a bridge between my mind and my body, a form of somatic meditation. In a complete reversal of my past attitude, I practice it as a meditational experience in the first place and as a physical exercise as a secondary goal. Nothing steadies my mind better than five - ten minutes of steadying my body in the balancing poses, whether they are upright poses, like tree or eagle asanas or inversions, like headstands or half-moon asana. Yoga finally became a conversation between my body and my mind.

I certainly was taught in the yoga classes before that pushing harder is not always the shortest path to the advancement of your skills, but it took me a while to truly accept it as my modus operandi. I am finally learning what was long known to the athletes, that by stressing less about the results and focusing more on being in the flow of the movement you can do more and better. It is quite like my running experience: The less I stress out over running faster, the better I perform.

Qi Gong
When my both hands were engulfed in neuropathic pain and crippled, most of yoga asanas became off limits for me. Then I thought of Qi gong. Qi gong is a Chinese form of healing arts based on the concept of Qi (the life source), much like acupressure, acupuncture and Chinese martial arts.

Kathleen, my acupressure teacher, teaches Qi gong both in the acupressure classes and as a stand-alone discipline. Too bad her classes could not fit into my schedule. So, I went online and found many videos with Qi gong routines. I picked the ones that were consistent with what I learned from Kathleen and started practicing Qi gong. I even memorized a couple of 10-minute routines that sustained me through my times away from yoga. Not as physically demanding as yoga, Qi gong may be better suited for those in chronic pain.

The healing benefits are similar because Qi gong, like yoga, engages the entire body. I found the slow and repetitive pace of Qi gong routines to be a great emotional stabilizer. Over time, my body memorized the routines and moved through them on autopilot, so my mind could relax in a meditative flow. I often played meditative tunes along with my practice ,and it helped to clear stress and refresh my mind. I still practice Qi gong and enjoy it greatly.

Overcoming Fear

Every person who took the TMS route to recovery can tell you their own tales of overcoming the fear. Fear of pain, fear of progressing debilitation, fear of losing medical insurance, fear of the unknown ahead.

My fear was so deep that I didn't need much experience in mindfulness to acknowledge its existence. My fear materialized in the image of Aunt Gina on my mind all the time. My first success in overcoming pain came after I started telling myself, repeatedly, that I had to overcome my fear if I wanted to heal.

That's when Amber Murphy, a pain psychologist from the LA Psychology Center, became my guardian angel. We talked every week for about two months, and all that time she kept at one thing: getting me out of my fear. It was around that time that I wrote a long farewell letter to my fear. It brought me some relief, but the actual farewell took months. Much like pain from a bad marriage does not end when a dissolution of marriage is recorded by the county clerk, my divorce from fear became final long after I wrote that letter.

My very important take away from talking to Amber and to other members of the TMS forum was that I learned, not on an intellectual level, but rather in my gut, that I am prone to worries and fears and I needed to adjust my mindset in how I react to the events of daily life.

I would be lying if I deny that it took me many months to stop being afraid of pain and dystonia. Dystonia scared me much more than pain. At least with pain, there were painkillers. They did not cure anything, but they brought me the much-needed temporary relief. I had many role models and solid support from TMS-ers on the forum who overcame chronic pain.

With dystonia, I was pretty much on my own. I believe I was the first member of the forum to recover from a persistent dystonia. Mainstream medicine has no known cure or relief for dystonia. Mine was vicious, and it was progressing. Everything I read and knew about dystonia spelled out a terrifying future of slow paralysis of the limbs, while there was no known cure. The more thought I put into coping with the situation, the more terrifying was the prospect of living. I could not help it but constantly thought how helpless I was going to become once I lose my ability to type, to cook, to brush my teeth, to walk, to get out of bed on my own....

But as I started meditating and exercising, I learned that it took my mind away from scary thoughts, and it also took my worries down a notch when the waves of fear came. My nervous system became more resilient to stress and worries. I started noticing the jittery state of mind early. Just as it would start rising, I made a deliberate effort to meditate in order to calm myself down. As I started noticing occasional small improvements in my condition, I started believing more and more that my condition was, in fact, reversible. My fear started slowly dissipating as I was gradually building up my faith in my ability to overcome dystonia.

Faith

I talk about faith in the *Cure vs. Healing* section, but I will repeat again and again: Faith is your key to recovery.

Being an agnostic by upbringing, I doubt everything, following Voltaire's maxim that "doubt is an uncomfortable position, certainty is absurd." I was educated in a firm belief in provable facts, science, and logic. I remember smiling sarcastically at the old wives' stories about miraculous recoveries of paralyzed people from laying on of hands. Back then, I knew for sure that it was utter nonsense. Laying hands had nothing to do with a real scientific practice. I doubted anything that was not proven by a scientific fact.

As I was struggling through the peaks of my desperation, I realized that there were no scientifically proven facts in my possession to hang on to. After all, the official medicine did not give me anything that looked logical or provable. The efficacy of official medicine was summed up by an NHS article: about 45% rate of noticeable relief in case of CTS. In case of CRPS, situation was even worse. Short of a miracle, there was no proven, science-based path to recovery. But I did not believe in miracles.

Dr. Sarno seemed to have some convincing statistics. However, his method put responsibility for recovery into my own hands. I needed to convince myself that I could live up to that responsibility and recover.

The problem was two-fold.

For one, I had doubts in Sarno's theory by itself since it did not have a stamp of approval from the FDA (looking back, I see some irony in my belief in the FDA but not in Sarno). But even if Sarno was right, all of his successes seemed to be with the patients whose symptoms were just pain, without evidence of irreparable damage to the nerves. I doubted whether Sarno's approach could be sufficiently applied to my crippled, swollen, hypersensitive, red, and painful hands. I doubted whether my damaged nerves could be revived. I could not find any evidence of recovery from such significant damage to the body as I had experienced. And Ines from the CRPS forum – the one who recovered by re-reading Sarno's book many times - was no longer active there to assure me. Lack of reassurance fueled my obsessive worries that maybe her condition was not as bad as mine, maybe she never had dystonia, maybe she didn't have swelling, maybe it was not in both limbs.... I could continue my list of doubts forever.

But secondly, since the miracle of recovery did not occur upon the first or even the second reading of the Sarno book, I doubted my own ability to find and successfully execute that yet-to-be-found mindbody prescription suitable for me. To make matters worse, I had no idea how to define that prescription. All I knew was that it had something to do with my emotional state and my nervous system – a needle in a haystack.

In my doubts, I was supported by an authoritative source, a high-achieving woman, Michelle Obama, who once said: "The one way to get me to work my hardest was to doubt me." I, too, always worked harder. In this case, the solution was to do the opposite, to stop working myself into the ground. if you got sick by overworking your mind and your body, work less or figure out how to rest properly! But then I didn't know how to relax. I had dealt with the challenges my entire life by doubting my ability to achieve the goals, so I would be motivated to work harder in overcoming a challenge.

This clearly was a catch-22: to motivate myself, I had to doubt, but to recover – I had to believe in myself and relax. In order to recover, I had to work hard on relaxing, but my obsessive desire to work hard on everything could have been a root of my problems to begin with.

In a nutshell, believing in myself and my abilities to overcome a challenge was not my thing. Every achievement in my life came as a surprise to me, after doing the hard work of trying to get there by the way of doubting myself. It was probably a subconscious intent to avoid disappointments in life, or a result of low self-esteem, or maybe just a plain superstition.

The more I contemplated my next moves, the more I realized that I had to change my attitude. But how do you change the attitude, which had become almost automatic, a habit, a behavioral norm?

This is when Dr. Claire Weekes [12] came to my rescue.

I found a link to her recordings on the TMS website. I played them and was mesmerized by her voice. Dead for 20 years, this amazing woman continued to help the scores of sufferers of chronic pain, severe anxiety, and debilitating depression.

I will never forget her voice, firm, decisive and kind at the same time, colored by a slight Aussie accent: "This is Doctor Weekes speaking. I am very happy to have this opportunity to talk to you personally. First, I want to say that however long you may have suffered from nervous illness, if you wish to recover – you can".

I played her recording hundreds of times. I read posts of my fellow TMSers online. I made a deliberate effort to start building up my faith in myself.

I started collecting stories of successful recoveries. One story made a lasting impression on me. A man was diagnosed with stage 4 cancer, with a chance of survival at about 5%. Despite gloomy prospects, he decided to join those in the 5% group, not the other 95%. He recovered. A skeptic would say that it was a random draw of luck. However, nobody would meet their luck without trying. At that time, I told myself that if he could make it into the lucky 5% of cancer patients, I should be able to make it into the lucky 20% of CRPS patients.

I started taking a notice of every little improvement and congratulated myself on every minor success. As my confidence grew, my faith in myself grew, and my fear started diminishing. I noticed that with every small reduction in pain and contraction of muscles, my mood became more optimistic. Optimism, in turn, increased my desire to meditate more, to exercise more, to seek more activities that were joyful.

While my hands, feet, and ankles were still in pain, I ventured onto my ritual summer backpacking trip to Sierra Nevada. I hoped that my pain would ease up if I could disconnect myself from the problems and stresses of everyday life. Isn't that why my back pain and migraines miraculously subsided during my prior backpacking trips? I thought that it would be a good test of Dr. Sarno's theory.

Backpacking is hard work, eight - twelve miles a day up and down hills with a heavy backpack on your back is not necessarily pleasant. But the rewards outweigh the hardships of arduous work. Breathtaking scenery, peaceful and majestic landscape, and swimming in pristine lakes always gave me a boost and rejuvenation for the year ahead. This time, hiking was harder than usual. My feet and ankles shot back with pain after every step, but I kept walking, although slower than usual. After the second night on the trail, my feet did not hurt anymore. By the third night, we reached the highest point of the trip, and the hardest part of the hike was behind us.

We set our camp near a beautiful blue lake surrounded by granite cliffs and pine trees. Clouds were gathering for the afternoon thunderstorm. Snow peaks were so close and so pristine! For once, I was happy.

Exhausted by a long hike, I slept very well that night. When I woke up in the morning, my hands were free of pain and tension. They felt almost normal for several hours. At that point, I knew that my mental state and my restless mind were behind my illness.

In the months to come, there were several times when tension in my hands lifted for a few minutes or even for several hours. Sometimes I could track it back to a specific prior event, but more often I could not explain why dystonia would disappear suddenly and then suddenly return. However, it was enough for me to dispel the myth of a permanent damage to my nerves and irreparable dystonia. I started believing that my emotional state was both the trigger of my illness and the key to recovery.

Feeling Stuck

Every person who has been able to successfully beat back chronic pain by using the mindbody approach is very familiar with the feeling of being stuck. This is how it goes. One goes through years of suffering from chronic pain, and, at the time of despair, discovers the TMS method. He/she has an epiphany: Yes, my personality is typical for a TMS-er: hardworking, uptight, worrier, perfectionist, highly responsible – and susceptible to chronic pain. Sounds promising, right? But then doubts kick in.

A recurring theme on the TMS forum was doubts. Doubts about the poster's chances for recovery and doubts about whether they do in fact have TMS. Even after people would see some improvement, they often fell into the state of despair. Questions were presented in various forms, but they all boiled down to the following calculations: I was doing better (or even great), but now suddenly my progress stopped (or even reversed). Is it because I am doing something wrong (or maybe because I just was not born to be free of pain)?

It is human nature to obsess, to focus, to worry, to fear. Those who were fortunate to be born on a different side of the spectrum, who live in the moment, worrying only about what happens today, not saving a buck for the future, not thinking about saying a wrong or offensive word, not feeling a hormonal rush of panic over scary things that may never happen anyway - they live their lives mostly pain free but facing other problems that we may never encounter.

This is what I wrote in September 2016, a year into my illness.

TMSers do not know how to not obsess, hence we obsess with our pains and our fears, which obviously inhibits the recovery.

About 3-4 months into my journey I realized that despite Sarno's reassurances that I would not need to change my lifestyle to recover and live a happy life, I still needed to change my lifestyle. For a reason that is very simple: I had no clue how to be happy in my life. If things are good, I start worrying that they will get worse. If things are bad, I worry that they will never get better or would get even worse.

If I am always worried, I can't heal from doing nothing. If I could, I would have recovered 7 months ago, upon my first round through Sarno's book. My struggles in the last few months have been about finding a balance between not thinking about TMS and just doing things despite TMS versus doing the same very things obsessively in order to overcome TMS. It is all about the intent that we put into our actions. If our intent is about living in the moment and enjoying those few symptom-free minutes without anxious thought that those minutes would not last long - we will heal. If we continue worrying that symptoms will re-appear - we will not.

Zillion times did I declare myself fear-free, only to find few minutes later that I am still a slave to my fears. A true TMS-er, I would chew myself up for fearing, for not recovering soon enough, for doing too little, for doing too much.

The truth is that we all are very different. We should not compare ourselves to others and use others' timelines as a benchmark or to even have a timeline of our own. It is not a competitive sport, it is a personal journey. It is all about how we arrive on conquering our fears and obsessions. The path could be through ignoring pain or through relaxing until it goes away, or through journaling or through crying our sorrows out on the shoulder of a TMS psychologist - but it is only when we learn how to let our fear, anxiety and worry pass through our system without disturbing our inner peace - we will reach the destination point.

It took me another long year to conclude that I was firmly on the path to recovery.

There were some changes that happened to me on my way. I finally started to understand Buddhism as a lifestyle. In my daily life, I started noticing my inner tension, something that had been a constant before. Unrelated to the events of the day, it was a tension generated by my restless mind, tension of feeling stuck.

The more I enjoyed meditation as a process of its own, not as a task from a recovery manual, the more I felt improvement in my symptoms. The more I learned how to relax into just being, just watching a glimmering surface of the pool on a sunny day, just swimming for the pleasure of swimming and not for the purpose of recovering - the better I did. I was learning how to forget about my worries for a moment while looking at the flowers or trees in the park, or simply enjoying

114

a small talk with a stranger in the street. And the more I tried, the longer my worry-free and pain-free moments were.

In the common TMS parlance, all of the above means that I became more outcome independent.

Non-Linear Recovery and Extinction Bursts

One of the most important things each TMS-er needs to learn and memorize well is that your recovery, unless you are one of the very few lucky exceptions, will not be linear. You will experience what Dr. Sarno called "extinction bursts," which are explosions of symptoms in random places. The explosions may or may not match your main symptoms. They may make you feel stuck and throw you back into the state of despair.

I dare to say that I do not agree with the explanation that Dr. Sarno gave to the cause of extinction bursts, but his observations and even the term itself match my experiences precisely.

For example, about four months into my recovery, I woke up one morning with a severe pain in my right upper back. Muscles in my neck, shoulder, and part of my back below the right shoulder blade were not only incredibly painful, but also locked up in a powerful contraction so strong that they felt paralyzed. I could not sit up in bed, had to roll onto my stomach, and then carefully slide down onto my knees on the floor near my bed. I could not use my right arm for at least an hour. Slowly, I was able to compose myself and started working through the muscles, stretching them one by one, until I was able to take a shower and get dressed. I was able to go to work that day, and by the end of the next day everything was nearly back to normal with my upper back. At first, I was terrified, but quickly remembered Dr. Sarno's warning and was emotionally prepared to deal with an extinction burst.

Extinction bursts masquerade themselves in various forms and shapes and can puzzle and scare even a very experienced TMS-er. Nearly two years into recovery, I was leaving a grocery store with a heavy bag in my left hand, when suddenly my left thumb tensed up, turned into a straight unbending stick, and started pulling toward the rest of my fingers, eventually resting on top of my index finger in a bizarrely unnatural twist. It surely looked broken or dislocated. The force of my tendons and ligaments was such that I could barely pull it back with my other hand. My forearm felt the tension almost all the way to the elbow.

By then, I knew well not to worry. Moreover, the less I worry, the sooner I can get over the burst. I sat down in the car, closed my eyes, and started meditating. It was not easy to concentrate on meditation in the noisy parking lot. Adding to the difficulty was that for a couple days prior, my anxiety levels were higher than normal (another sign of extinction burst!), but after about five minutes of meditation, my thumb slowly relaxed and travelled back into its place. I drove safely home and soon forgot about this little incident. Had it happened to me earlier, in my less TMS-educated times, I would have been scared and fed on my fear for days after the incident.

For a while, on and off, I was getting quite bad and painful muscle cramps in my legs. I had never been prone to muscle cramps before. I quickly understood that muscle cramps were just another form of extinction bursts. Yet, driven by panic and information from medical websites, I asked my doctor to give me a referral to test the level of magnesium in my body. Even before the test results from the lab were back, the cramps disappeared. Tests showed normal levels of magnesium. I laughed at myself and slowly learned what to do about cramps. When a cramp attack happens, I try to relax the muscles, go into a meditation, and breathe. It helps much faster than twisting or shake my cramped limb in frustration or getting upset and worried. Believe me, I've tried it both ways.

One extinction burst was especially difficult. As pain in my wrists started receding about four months into recovery, it reappeared in my arms and legs. After a while, a dull, continuous pain spread into the buttocks and upper back, and I started to suspect that I had developed fibromyalgia. This one lasted for several very long months and was quite difficult for me emotionally and physically, since my energy level dropped again. I started to fear that I was losing my battle with CRPS and was acquiring yet another incurable illness. Fortunately, after a while, this dull, unending muscle pain started slowly going away and completely disappeared about six months later.

Anxiety and depression are very common conditions for those with TMS. Our personalities lend themselves to both emotional disorders. Be prepared to see a rise in anxiety and/or depression during extinction bursts, even if you consider yourself generally free of both. They are an emotional mirror of your pain symptoms and are inexplicably linked to your chronic pain, your muscle spasms – and however else your TMS is manifesting itself.

One may ask a question: How do I distinguish between an extinction burst and a permanent worsening of my condition? It is a complicated question that I can only answer with confidence for my specific case. I experienced dozens of sudden rises in symptoms, specifically in pain level, muscle spasms, anxiety, and depression. I would be lying if I claimed that it never worried me. I panicked many times, especially when symptoms persisted for more than two - three days.

Eventually I learned not to panic – see more in the section *Faith*.

Much harder than extinction bursts were plateaus, maybe because they were not explicitly mentioned in Dr. Sarno's book.

Plateau

As I moved through my recovery, each extinction burst was followed by a slight improvement in symptoms and then a plateau, when progress seemed to stop. A plateau could last for a month or six months. During those times, I did not see any improvement. Those were the hardest.

After a few months of anxiously waiting for any progress, I would start to worry. What if it would never get better? What if I would forever depend on Topricin to make the fire ants stop crawling through my hands? What if I would be forever stuck not being able to write my signature, let alone a birthday card, to hold my hand flat against the table, to shake hands with people, to snap my fingers? Would I be ever able to do a handstand again?

As I put timeline of my recovery together, I noticed that those plateaus coincided with the irrational things that I did. It was during those plateaus that I signed up for expensive, yet useless treatments that I did not need and tried various vitamins and diets. And each time, after a few days or weeks, I would calm down, and unfinished bottles of food supplements would become another casualty of my anxiety over my illness.

As I write this chapter, I am in the longest plateau to date. It has been at least ten months since I recorded my last noticeable improvement, being able to snap fingers on my right hand. The prior longest plateau was almost five months, after fingers on my left hand finally produced a perfect snap at the end of July 2017. While in the plateau, I was able to finally get into a handstand, increased number push-ups I could do without resting to 20-25 and returned to my normal lifestyle – meaning that dystonia is no longer front and center of my daily experiences. In TMS-speak, not worrying about achieving full recovery is called outcome independence.

My hands are back to the level of dexterity before CRPS, but they are still a bit puffy and my middle fingers still feel slightly numb. I can't help it, but every once in a while, I get concerned whether they will ever close that 1% gap to perfection. I wonder if I will get to the point that I no longer care about whether I have the symptoms or not - maybe then I will recover 100%?

Frozen Emotions

The cornerstone of Sarno's psychological approach is to find the source and the cause of what he calls a rage. It is your suppressed anger, caused by unsatisfied desires, unfulfilled ego, neglected self. Rage, per Sarno, causes emotional and physical pain and turns up as pain and tension in unexpected places like your back or neck. But if suppressed anger can do that to you, why not other suppressed emotions?

I always believed that people must fully control their emotions in a professional environment, no matter what. Spilling your emotions on unsuspecting coworkers or neighbors is wrong. Crying openly over your personal dramas at work is unprofessional – that's what I always believed. It is especially unacceptable for the bosses in a bad mood to take it out on their subordinates.

And that's what I did in my life. I took it even one step further. Even in tragic circumstances, I didn't let emotions out at work. I did not allow myself to cry. I did not allow myself to be open about my grief even with myself. Believing that I needed to stay strong, I pushed my emotions inside. Tears came many months later, but only during sleepless nights. They did not bring any relief.

As I was reading Dr. Sarno's book, it occurred to me that this had been the way I dealt with my emotions along my life path. Through many trying times, my way of handling hardships was to not show even to myself how scared or sad I was. Shame was the only emotion I did not know how to overcome or push inside. Worry was the only emotion that I allowed to run its course freely – it seemed to be a practical one, it encouraged my problem solving and prompted my search for Plan B and all the way to Plan Z, to get all the bases covered.

By my late 30s, I stopped crying. I still remembered how, as a child, I used to cry until there was no more sorrow inside me. I decided that not crying meant being a grown-up. "Big girls do not cry" – I told myself. I still had tears of compassion while watching a movie or a play, but not for myself. It was lost on me that, in addition to negative emotions, my positive emotions also disappeared. I stopped feeling joy, excitement, and even curiosity. My life became a journey through responsibilities. I became a task handler.

Looking back, I wonder if the way I dealt with my emotions throughout my adult life led me to the severe outburst of rosacea within weeks of my mother's death and to developing CRPS a few months after my father died? CRPS encroached on me slowly, with my shoulders, knees, and ankles getting tighter and tighter, with insomnia and migraines hitting harder and harder by late summer of 2015. And then – all the past stresses must have caught up with me, and a floodgate opened a couple months later and resulted in CRPS and dystonia.

Something that I noticed as a sign of frozen emotions was my response to music. Devoid of any abilities to make music, I enjoy listening very much. Or, to be precise, I enjoyed listening to music very much until my emotions froze completely a couple of years before CRPS hit. Slowly, I migrated from enjoying music to crossing out items on my cultural to-do list. I would listen to the music and imagine how I should be feeling at this time. I could not understand why music was not as emotionally intense or rewarding to me anymore – until I realized that I had emptied out my emotional reserves.

This is what I wrote in the spring of 2016, while trying to find the source of my pain in the depth of my unconscious:

Unfortunately, my response to all the challenges of life had been to push my feelings aside and plow my way through, with migraines, chronic fatigue, depression, anxiety, back pain, neck and shoulder pain being my life-long companions. Result? Pain there, emotions are gone, including joy, excitement, pleasure.... I often "tell" myself how to feel, knowing that in the past I used to feel this and that on a similar occasion. I used to be an emotional person - but I am feeling emotionally flat, even though people tell me that I am a warm person. They may feel the warmth of my personality - but I don't. Stuck and can't figure out what to do.

A lot of our bad emotional hygiene comes from restrictive social norms and expectations that we should control our emotions. I still agree with that. But what should we do in the situations where emotions arise, yet, must be controlled and not spilled on people around us?

There is a way. I took a class on how to handle negative emotions from a Buddhist educational center. In the class, I learned how to walk my negative emotions through the physical sensations in my body and how to release them: fear, anger, sadness, and anxiety alike. After all, our emotions are directly connected to our hormonal system. Emotions arise in our mind, but they have their direct counterparts in our body. It is better to "feel through" the negative emotion physiologically - than push it into subconscious and set yourself up for emotional and physical pain.

In my healing journey, the more I meditated, the more I found that my emotions were coming back. The class that I took on emotions gave me the tools to recognize my emotions and notice how my mind quickly and routinely pushes them into the subconscious. I learned that emotions are part of what we are, and that we, humans, find negative emotions unpleasant and unbearable, so we do our best to hide from the unpleasant feelings.

I started with sitting meditation in full silence. At some point, I discovered that very monotonous chanting was helping me to concentrate. Eventually, I started replacing my usual monotonous and rhythmic meditation tunes with the ones that were more emotionally colored. Of the tunes that I picked out of the treasure trove of YouTube, a special mention should go to the Tina Turner channel.

Tina made a surprising transition from her stardom in pop and rock to Buddhist chanting and singing. Her chanting invariably brings me to tears and releases my emotions, the ones that I otherwise so skillfully push inside, where they simmer in subconscious and cause me physical pain.

After two years of meditation and focus on my emotional hygiene, I noticed the return of my emotions.

Unfortunately, emotions came back at a cost because my anxiety returned, too. I am not the only one to experience a return of an emotional disorder as soon as my physical symptoms started fading away. Other members of the TMS community reported a rise in depression and/or anxiety after their chronic pain was gone.

I am not happy about the return of anxiety and depression, but I am much more mindful about it now. I understand that by pushing my emotions away or deeply inside my mind, I am activating some pain pathways in my brain. Being able to feel them through is extremely important, no matter how unpleasant or painful it may be. The upside is that I now feel my beloved mountain landscapes and music again, in an emotional way.

I still maintain my emotional composure with others. I do not let myself down by spilling my negative emotions on others at work, but I've learned to recognize my emotions as they come and not allow them to drop into my subconscious.

How do I deal with anxiety and depression? I sense the onset of those anxiety waves and use my newly acquired knowledge to process my emotions: acknowledge them, let them run their course no matter how unpleasant they are, feel sadness, anxiety, anger, or fear – whatever comes my way. I know that those emotions, no matter how strong they are, are relatively short-lived and that a better day will come. Often, I take three - five minutes for a short meditation if I feel anxious in a stressful situation.

I can't say that I am 100% successful at closing every emotional page in the book of my life. But this is who I am. I know that my nervous system is overly sensitive and is susceptible to the impact of the external forces and I need to learn how to absorb and process the impact without causing myself physical pain. I keep trying, work in progress.

Dr. Render, Osteopath

Summer of 2016 was eventful and overwhelming. I was about five months into the TMS journey. Neuropathic pain in my hands was mostly gone, but it was replaced by a new kind of pain. It was milder, widespread, and it came with a debilitating fatigue. It was a dull, never-ending pain that rarely got much better or much worse, and it was concentrated in my upper arms, elbows, shoulders and around my knees and ankles. It was always there, day or night.

My symptoms clearly resembled fibromyalgia, another form of TMS described by Dr. Sarno. I kept meditating and journaling, but the pain was not going away. During that long plateau in the summer of 2016, I became worried. What if it is not an extinction burst? What if my pain is not fibromyalgia or TMS? What if I am not doing it right? What if I am not one of those 20% of Sarno's patients who would take a long, but finite time to recover; instead, what if I am a hopeless deadbeat, unaccounted for by Dr. Sarno's statistics?

Now, looking back, I know with certainty that it was just another extinction burst and subsequent plateau, but back then I was too inexperienced in dealing with TMS.

Fibromyalgia symptoms were so unpleasant that I started searching for other ways out of pain. I came across a book by Dr. Andrew Weil, *Spontaneous Recovery*. The book described many cases of spontaneous recovery from various illnesses that could not be explained by the mainstream medicine. A couple of chapters of his book were dedicated to his friend, an osteopathic physician responsible for several unexplained recoveries of otherwise incurable patients. Anxious for a quick solution, one more time I decided to look for somebody to "fix" me.

I remembered that a friend told me about her primary physician, Dr. Render, who was practicing osteopathy, unlike many DOs who switched completely to general medicine. My phone conversation with Dr. Render was not reassuring. She has had some very good results with IBS (irritable bowel syndrome) patients, but she never had patients like me. She agreed to give it a try but promised nothing beyond her best effort. I had little to lose and switched to her as my primary physician.

I checked in Sarno's book after our phone call. IBS was listed as a possible TMS condition, so I felt that there was promise. The extra challenge was that her office was almost 30 freeway miles away – and I could not drive that far anymore. My otherwise 35-minute drive to see her was planned with all the necessary contingencies, for a total of 1.5 hours. I stopped several times on the way to rest when the neuropathic pain increased and fire ants started crawling through my hands, but I was very proud of myself for being able to make that trip!

Dr. Render, a young petite woman with a radiant smile, was all kindness and attention. I decided that, osteopathy aside, having a caring and open-minded family physician was worth the exhausting drive.

Neither one of us had grand expectations, as we both knew that she was taking a path of trial and error. In the beginning of each session, she would explain what her plan was and whether she would try something new. A day or two after the session, I would usually email her a status update.

After initial unsuccessful attempts to work directly on my hands and arms, Dr. Render switched her attention to my head and neck, maybe following the clues from Dr. Sarno's theory or maybe consistent with the approach that she took with her IBS patients. We both felt that results could have been better if she could see me weekly, but she had a very busy schedule, so I came on average once a month for about a year.

Not right away, but gradually, interesting things started happening. Each time, Dr. Render was making changes in her routine and finally arrived onto something that made a difference. She started sessions with the area above and to the left of my navel. She explained that in her IBS patients that area was always tender. Interestingly, it was quite painful in me initially, too, but became less and less sore over time. After attending to the belly, she would move to my head. As she gently touched my head, neck, and chest, making small, almost undetectable movements, I would feel a surge of emotions - sometimes very subtle, sometimes stronger. Sometimes, my legs or arms, or even my entire body would twitch unexpectedly. I do not remember any twitching in the early sessions, but it happened more frequently toward the end.

Nothing changed in my symptoms on the day of the visit. But then, the next day I noticed that the hold of dystonia on me would ease up a bit, for an hour or so. Then my hands would lock up again, but those couple hours of improvement energized our determination to continue.

One day, in February 2017, Dr. Render had a trainee with her, a student from the local school of osteopathy. She herself was doing her usual routine, while the student was tasked with working on my hip area. As they were working on me, something shifted in my emotional state. I can't explain it well, but it felt like an emotional shake-up. But the real shake-up came the next day. This is what I wrote to her in my status report:

> *Just wanted to give you an update: after the last visit, something extraordinary happened. After about 26 hours of increased anxiety and depressive feelings (which is quite common after the treatment), I, all of a sudden, experienced a nearly complete release of tension in both wrists and hands. It was a bliss! My left wrist has been free of blockage for a while, but right wrist was quite tense. The release lasted for about 5-6 hours and then blockage returned, but I know it was just a beginning. I am excited!*

The release in tension was similar to what I had experienced during my backpacking trip six months earlier, but deeper and longer. The return of the tension was not as gradual as back in the mountains. It was almost like a flip of a switch.

We were never able to replicate that effect, whether with a student assistant, or without. Still, by the end of August 2017, I was doing well enough to end my visits. She was in great demand by the chronic pain patients, and they needed her more than I did.

I now see her about once a year, for my physical – an easy patient for a busy family doctor!

Dr. Farias

Around the same time that I started talking to Dr. Render, I came across the website of Dr. Joaquin Farias, a neuroscientist from the University of Toronto. It gave me the first indication that dystonia was not a dead-ended condition and could be beaten.

Dr. Farias himself experienced dystonia as a professional pianist at age 21, but recovered from it, being guided by inquisitive mind, intuition, and determination. Dystonia naturally became his area of scientific research. In addition to his research, he started conducting workshops for the dystonia patients, showing them in practice how they could heal themselves from dystonia.

I will not go into the details of his theory and experience teaching people how to re-wire their brains and heal from dystonia – he wrote a book (*Limitless - How Your Movements Can Change Your Brain*), which presents it very eloquently in a language quite accessible for a non-scientist. Instead, I will describe my own experiences at his workshop, which I attended in October 2016.

There were three of us in the workshop: a woman who stopped using her hand due to hypotonia (reduced muscle tonus), a young software engineer whose fingers frequently stumbled on the computer keyboard while otherwise doing just fine, and me, whose wrists and hands had a persistent hyper tonus of the muscles. I was the only one who had neuropathic pain in addition to dystonia.

In a way, the workshop was similar to the lectures by Dr. Sarno, but by far more neuroscience-infused and aided by many practical exercises to learn and take home to practice. He explained the mechanism of dystonia and how the brain induces it.

Dr. Farias confirmed what I already believed: My problems were not local to my hands; they were originating in my brain and were of a psychosomatic nature. He neither explicitly confirmed, nor denied the emotional factor as a root cause of my problem, but he strongly underscored the importance of meditation, yoga, and other energy-based healing arts for recovery. It was very important to me as it re-assured me that I was on the right path.

But he also taught me other very important things. He had me use my less affected right hand to unbend my fingers on my left hand - a simple trick that I may have done unconsciously before but never took a serious note of. My fingers straightened out, although with pain. Then, forced by the other hand, they as easily folded into a loose fist. You see – he said – your tendons are just fine, they can do it, the problem is in the brain.

He also explained that dystonia is unlikely to originate on both sides of the body. The other side is just a mirror. He advised me to focus on my left hand as the most affected. The most important recommendation from him was not to be afraid to force your muscles out of the dystonic grip. In my case, he wanted me to force my left hand into the fist. On the first day of the workshop, I tried really hard, until my pain became unbearable. Once I stopped pressing – my left hand went back, right where it was before. Clearly, I had more work to do.

On my last morning in Toronto, I went for a walk in the park and decided to try again. As used as I was to the strange behavior of my brain, I was very surprised by what happened next. I used my less affected right hand to press my left hand into a fist. I pressed harder and harder, bending my wrist to add to the pressure, despite the pain, pins and needles piercing my hand and arm. At some point, it felt as if I was holding a bare electric wire, and electric current was flowing through my hand, wrist and forearm, culminating in an explosion of pain and what felt like strong electric shock throughout my hand and wrist.

Scared, I let go of my hand, and pain and shock were gone. But also gone was the tension in my wrist and thumb. It was now gripping only a part of my hand, from the crease of the palm to the tips of my fingers, mostly the middle and index fingers, but the grip was much weaker than before. My left wrist has been tension-free since.

But another interesting thing happen. My right hand, which was supposed to be a mere mirror, decided to take an independent role and got a little worse, just confirming another of Dr. Farias's assertion that every case of dystonia is unique. The negative shift in the right hand was not nearly as dramatic as the positive shift in the left hand and did not alter my victorious mood. I knew I was on the path to recovery.

Three hours later, at the workshop, Dr. Farias commented on my success story that since my dystonia developed on top of neuropathic pain, it would likely be going out with the pain. It was consistent with my prior experiences of extinction bursts – explosions of pain – preceding every small improvement in my symptoms. I was ready to endure more pain but rid myself of dystonia.

There was also another confirmation of the emotional underpinning of my dystonia. At the end of the workshop, Dr. Farias brought in a set of sensors to produce an EEG brain image on his computer. We watched what happened in the brain of the software engineer as his fingers were stumbling while he was typing on the keyboard, and Dr. Farais explained how the brain functioning was impacting the ability of his hands to perform the movements. Then it was my turn. I wanted to test how my emotions arise in response to music. I asked to put on my most favorite piece of music by Bach, which used to bring me to tears before I became sick.

At the end of the class, I received a video of my brain responding to Bach. The left side of my brain, ultimately responsible for processing the music, was barely activated. Dr. Farias explained that it could be because the piece was so well imprinted in my memory, my brain was just focused on the memory recall - and this is what lit up the right side of my front lobe. But that confirmed my other suspicion – I still had a lot of meditation to do in order to unfreeze my emotions. Two years later, I would love to repeat the EEG of my brain while listening to the music – would my left brain respond better now?

Acupressure and Qi
In the fall of 2016, I also restarted acupressure sessions, now on a regular basis with my friend Panda. When we started,

she told me that to her, my wrists and hands "felt like a block of concrete."

I must add some explanations for those who are not familiar with Chinese medicine. Chinese medicine's definition of Qi can be loosely translated into our Western terms of "life source" or "energy." Some authors [14] make an analogy between Qi and electric signals that run through our nervous system. Remember Dr. W and his verdict, that nerves in my wrists stopped conducting electric signals? A trained practitioner of Chinese medicine, Panda did not need an EMG to come to a similar conclusion. She "felt" the flow of Qi. What she described as "blockage" of Qi, was probably manifesting itself through the blockage of electrical signals.

Since my own acupressure training stopped at the beginner level, I never progressed enough to be able to consistently detect Qi in other people – something that experienced practitioners do almost unconsciously. So, I was left to admire that whatever Panda's fingers were reporting back to her matched closely my own sensations of constraint and pressure in my wrists and hands, which felt very real and physical, as if my hands and wrists were filled with a mix of sand and epoxy. Yes, "a mix of sand and epoxy" is as close as I can define the sensation during those times. As a matter of fact, I could clearly and consistently identify the border between the impacted and healthy parts of my wrist. When I pressed my left hand into the fist in Toronto and felt a shockwave, the amount of the "epoxy sand" in my hand shrank instantly after.

As the sensations of constraint and pressure were gradually shrinking over time, first out of my wrists, then out of the palms of my hands, and eventually out of my fingers, my hands became lighter, more flexible and less "foreign." On her end, Panda was feeling that Qi slowly started flowing to my fingers.

At the time of writing, the sensation of constraint and mild numbness persists only in the tip of my left middle finger and on the inside of my right middle finger and a small area of the palm of my hand adjacent to middle finger. It is the last remaining puffy spot on my hand that reminds me of how swollen my hands were less than two years ago. The tension is no longer powerful enough to force the contraction of my ligaments. I have a full control of my both hands, and minor discomfort does not prevent me from going about my normal life.

Panda and I worked together to devise an acupressure routine that focused on stress relief. Often, as Panda was gently calming down my nervous system, my body responded with a sudden twitch and then emotional release, very similar to how it responded during Dr. Render's sessions. I find it quite remarkable that the Five Elements theory of Chinese medicine explains very convincingly a connection between my personality type and the impact of stress on my mind and body, which resulted in the strain on my muscles and joints.

In addition to gently balancing my nervous system, Panda provided me with her observations of how my body was changing with time. With ups and downs, the general direction was toward gradual improvement. Together, we celebrated every little ability returning to my hands, whether it was being able to write, or make a fist, or snap my fingers, or get into the handstand. Needless to say, Panda no longer feels the "block of concrete" in my wrists and hands.

Support Team

In this section, I will repeat what is well known to many survivors of terrible illnesses like cancer, stroke, or heart attack: You cannot fight your serious health condition on your own. You need a support team.

Every person mentioned in the foreword became part of my support team – knowingly or unknowingly. Without them, I would have never made it this far.

Your support team can be your doctors, or your family, or your friends, or your fellow patients, or even strangers – or all the above. Make sure that each time you interact with somebody with regards to your medical condition, you assess how helpful they are to the course you have chosen. It does not mean that anyone who questions your chosen course of action should be ignored or dismissed.

Maybe because of my professional background, I tend to welcome questioning of my ideas and plans. It helps me to clarify and adjust my course of action. You should keep your mind open and consider every option that comes your way, but every option should be examined with scrutiny and assessed on the merits it would offer to your individual case. We all are unique, and what worked for someone else may not work for you.

I looked at and discarded many alternative treatments and methods that were discussed on the TMS forum. It does not make those treatments less valuable for others. It only means that they were not working for me. Likewise, I stayed with other practitioners and their methods as I found them helpful to me.

Often more important than methods were the practitioners themselves. I was lucky to find Amber and Alan, the pain psychologists. I only spoke to Alan once, for three minutes, but his courses posted on the TMS Wiki became my daily read and practice for many months. I became emotionally connected to both. I am certain that Alan does not remember a brief conversation I had with him – but I do. He is a big part of my support team because even now I read his essays and posts and learn new things. I already wrote about Amber, who became my cheerleader and was kind and generous enough to stay in touch with me after her paid work was over.

A big part of my support team were people from the TMS forum. They were compassionate and incredibly patient as they answered my questions and gave me much-needed encouragement. Any time I was in a desperate mood, somebody on the forum would respond to my plea for help, right at the time I needed it. Thank you, TMSers!

I was very lucky to find Dr. Render and have her as my family doctor. She is a thoughtful, intelligent, caring, and courageous physician. My visits with her had osteopathic treatments as a primary goal but also helped me to put a structure around my chaotic process of trial and error. Could I have made it without a primary doctor like her? Possibly – but it would have taken me much longer time and much more work on my own.

Prior close ties with a person are not an unconditional qualification for them to join your support team. Even within my familial and friendship circles, not everyone became part of my team. They may have not been a fit into the roles I needed so much at the times of desperation, which absolutely does not make them any less dear to my heart, and they still all remain my beloved family and friends.

Some people entered my support team briefly and unknowingly, like the yoga teacher who gently helped me to get into a handstand. She did not know that less than a year prior I could not even put the palms of my hands flat on the floor and was told not to put any pressure on my wrists. We met briefly, but I have the fondest memories of her – she helped me to let go of my fear. Another member of my team was my physical therapist Leigh, who kept telling me that she could no longer be helpful to me after completing first eight sessions. She likely didn't understand that her kindness and compassion kept me afloat through the worst times and meant much more to my survival than her physical therapy instructions.

There were also people like my dear friends Panda and Kathleen whose acupressure sessions not only helped me to get better, but also were delivered with a healthy dose of therapeutic encouragement at the time when I needed it so much. And, of course, I am forever grateful to Kathleen who recommended Dr. Sarno's book to me, which changed my life.

I came to believe that having a support team is an absolute requirement for healing. Somebody who believes in your ability to overcome the challenges that your body and your mind present to you.

As I think of every member of my support team, including long-deceased Dr. Weekes and Dr. Sarno, a warm feeling that fills my heart continues to heal my nervous system.

Journaling

Journaling is one of the techniques highly recommended by the TMS psychologists. I tried. As a daily practice, it did not work out well for me. Instead of relieving my stress, it increased it, as I obsessed over producing a complete meaningful essay every day. It had to be a story or otherwise I would be stuck in the writer's block, which happened pretty much every day. I never learned to dump my stream of consciousness on paper and out of my brain in a way that would ease my stress.

Eventually, I gave up on journaling in a recommended form and replaced the daily journaling practice with an occasional status report or an email to somebody about my condition. Instead of using journaling as a tool for psychoanalysis, I used my writing as a tool for summarizing my improvements, discussing my next steps with myself, and even as a mere way to encourage myself and to celebrate my achievements.

Even today, as I am spending at least a few hours every week writing this book, I feel how writing about my experience makes me more introspective and mindful. I keep looking back at the path I traveled and forward at the path ahead of me.

The advice that I can give on journaling is simple: Even if you don't succeed at it in the way you initially expected, don't give up. Writing is another exercise in mindfulness, introspection, and self-awareness. Some may find it a pretty good anti-anxiety pill – at least I often do. If you look at it in that way, it could be easier to put it to good use.

Encouragement, Reassurance, and Celebration

As I mentioned before, being chronically ill is a very lonely experience. It shrinks your universe and slowly dries out your contacts with people. A chronically ill person can reach out to other chronically ill people, but they frequently are sad companions, so you will be stuck in the doom and gloom. You need to learn how to become your own cheerleader.

I learned to look for encouragement everywhere. Each tiny improvement in symptoms I took as a confidence builder and a chance to celebrate and remind myself that I was getting better. This is what I wrote to Amber on Thanksgiving of 2016:

In my journey through pain, disability and despair, I found something that I can be thankful for. As a matter of fact, many things.

Thanksgiving holiday never meant this much to me. Yes, it was a day to get together with the family, to try to eat less, to stay away from the stores the following day when America rejoices in shopping. This time, it is truly a day of thanksgiving for me, as I am finally feeling that I am recovering, although I still have long ways to go.

I woke up this morning, feeling grateful. It used to be pain that woke me up. Now, I can sleep and not feel pain. I still feel pain most of the time during the day, but I know how to deal with it and I know that one day it will stop bothering me at all.

I have been living with dystonia and severe chronic pain for over a year. As a matter of fact, I realized that I had a milder form of it most of my life. My muscles and tendons were always tight, as my body was always in the fight-flight response, feeling the tiger behind my back, ready to spring into escape. Time to unlearn the fear – and it is an incredibly liberating experience.

I used to exercise out of fear that one day I would grow old, fat, crippled. My inner bully yelled at me to go and exercise. I am learning now how to experience a joy of feeling my body, feeling the pleasure of running, swimming, yoga. Now that I know what held me back: my fear of life.

I grew up poor and lived paycheck to paycheck until my mid 40-ies. I was always extremely tight with money and worried that tomorrow there will be no money to pay the bills. I am quite surprised to notice that I am less fearful of my financial standing. I am more likely to write a check to a charity, give a buck to a street beggar or buy a spontaneous gift to a friend. Not because I hit a jackpot or got a raise, but simply because I am less fearful of life. And I have my newly found understanding of my TMS to thank for it.

My parents were non-religious: mother an atheist, father only occasionally religious. I have been a reluctant agnostic all my adult life, but I am so thankful to TMS that it woke up my desire to learn things beyond discovered facts, beyond accepted scientific dogmas, beyond common knowledge. My desire to learn the language of faith.

I never felt as connected to myself and my body as I am now. Whether I meditate or not, I often take a minute in the middle of a busy day to say thank you to my limbs that still work, my heart that still beats, my lungs that still breathe. I came to understand what many people don't: that a debilitating pain comes with life and that power of mind frees us from that pain.

Phobias

As I continued on my path of meditation, mindfulness, and introspection, I confronted my fears many times. One of those times was when I admitted to myself that I had phobias. Even before that discovery, I was quite aware that I had a fear of heights. I also concluded long ago that fast driving, especially on the mountain roads, was not my forte.

Both fears, of height and speed, did not sit well with my love for the mountains, since my fears often kicked in exactly when I had to drive on the steep curvy roads to the trailheads, and even more so when I had to turn around on a hike, with a peak being within my reach, all for the fear of making those last 100 feet to the top!

While I fought my insomnia, anxiety, and life stresses in the years leading up to dystonia and CRPS, my phobias got worse. I became more and more cautious on the mountain roads, tall winding overpasses; more and more often I slowed down where other cars were going 60 miles an hour. Interestingly, it was a specific type of a road curve but not many other ones that caused my breathing to halt, my hands to sweat, my heart to start pounding – that's when the fear would overtake my normally rational mind. CRPS added surges of neuropathic pain to the already disturbing feelings of fear during those moments. I was terrified, in pain, and at the same time ashamed that I could not overcome my fear. That, in turn, exacerbated my fear.

But it was only now, with pain and dystonia in focus, that I consciously confronted my phobias in a way I have never tried before. I understood that anxiety and fear were interconnected, I started preparing myself to face my anxiety and my fears even before they kicked in. To fight my fears, I needed to bring down the level of anxiety and jitteriness that had become a constant presence in my mind and in my body. And the only way to do it reliably was mindfulness and meditation. I became better at recognizing my condition and being prepared to overcome the fears now, by de-sensitizing my nervous system.

I am still working on my fear of driving fast over the curves. I am finally back to driving on the overpasses that I avoided for almost three years. I am still driving in a slow lane, but I am able to overcome my fear. Work in progress.

Chapter 6. Summary

Timeline

To make it easier for the reader to have a quick grasp of my story, I put together my timeline. It is important for the reader to understand that when I started following Dr. Sarno's method, I expected to fully heal in three months. In reality, it took me more than two long years, and my recovery was not linear at all. Pain was gone relatively quickly, but dystonia proved to be much more resistant.

If you are trying to heal from a chronic pain and/or dystonia, pay attention to the extinction bursts and plateaus. It is important that you are aware of them and do not get discouraged. Knowing about those from Dr. Sarno's book and from the TMS forum helped me get through very difficult times when I thought that permanent improvement would never come.

Dates	Events	Symptoms
September 2015		Left hand and wrist swollen, painful, middle finger curled in
September 2015	First diagnosis	Carpal Tunnel Syndrome Diagnosis
November 2015	Vacation	Left hand and wrist swollen, painful, middle fingers curled in both hands. Neuropathic pain intensifies
December 2015		Lost ability to write Neuropathic pain in shoulders, arms, hands
January 2016	Learned about CRPS	Lost ability to drive more than 5-7 miles Hypersensitivity to

142

		temperature and touch Dystonia increases and persists in nearly all my fingers.
February 2016	Dr. Sarno's book	Dystonia is much worse
March 2016	Start of a plateau, ~ 1 month	Sleep improves significantly Some reduction in pain levels Increase in dystonia
April 2016	Extinction burst	Increase in pain Pain spreads to entire body
May 2016	Start of a plateau ~ 1 month	
June 2016	Started meditation	Some reduction in pain levels
July 2016	Extinction burst Start of a plateau	New pain - fibromyalgia-like fatigue
August 2016	Hiking in the mountains	Instant improvement in both hands, lasting for several hours. Then symptoms return
August 2016	First osteopathic session with Dr. Render Plateau continues	
October 2016	Workshop with Dr. Farias	Instant, lasting release in the left hand, dystonia intensifies in the right hand
October 2016	Start of plateau ~ 3	

143

	months	
December 2016	Resumed gentle yoga	Reynaud's symptoms are mostly gone
January 2017	Extinction burst	Frequent severe cramps in legs, feet, arms, continuing for at least 4 months
April 2017	Half-marathon in 2.5 hours! Start of a plateau ~3 months	
July 2017		Pain and tension in the left hand remains only in the middle finger, but I can snap fingers and the sound is solid and loud!
November 2017	Resumed full-scale yoga practice	Residual pain and stiffness in knees and ankles. Moderate dystonia in hands remains at night, but disappears in the morning
December 2017		Pain and tension in the right hand is down, enough for me to snap fingers on my right hand.
February 2018	Handstand!	Full dexterity in hands returned, both day and night. I no longer have a persistent dystonia, although on occasion I experience spasms and night-time spikes in pain and tension in my hands.
Summer 2018	The End	Cramps are gone. No night-time pain. Some minor

144

		numbness, mostly in the right hand, remains but does not bother me.

What I Learned

My story is coming to an end. But my life continues.

My experience did not change who I am. It made me more aware of who I am and who I am not. It aligned my self-image with my reality.

I learned that swatting away fears is cowardly, while confronting emotions, fears, and weaknesses is an act of true courage. I stopped lying to myself that I am a superhuman, even when I believe I need to be one.

I know that both my body and my mind, or more accurately, my mindbody, needs rest and maintenance. My agile and sensitive nervous system is my asset and the engine behind my accomplishments in life, but it is also my weakness. I learned how important it is for me to practice meditation in various forms, to watch my emotional state, and to balance out my weaknesses.

I learned that physical exercise is an absolute requirement for me, and I must exercise if I want to keep my mindbody in balance. My muscles and joints get stale and my mind irritable and restless if I don't. I continue to use all the tools I described in Chapter 5: mindfulness, meditation, yoga, running, Qi gong.

I am not alone in my self-realization. Many people who succeed in overcoming severe chronic pain and other neurological conditions meditate on a regular basis, keep their journals, and repeat online courses that Alan Gordon puts out so generously on the TMS Wiki.

If you want your car to work reliably and last longer, you take it to the mechanic for a tune-up and maintenance. If you want your mindbody to work reliably and last longer, you must tune it up on a regular basis – and it has to be mostly do-it-yourself. There is no magic pill. Each time I tried to throw money at my illness by buying expensive treatments, I learned repeatedly that magic pills do not exist – unless I put my own elbow grease into getting better by meditating or exercising.

Self-awareness and self-care will pay off in less pain and fewer visits to the doctors - at least to the back, neck, shoulder, and foot doctors. Because instead of treating the symptoms in your individual body parts, you will be keeping your entire self in balance and harmony.

Is a Complete Recovery Possible?

I know that many people have reported a complete, absolute recovery from chronic pain and moved on with their lives.

In full disclosure, I can't claim that I have recovered 100%. I am at about 99%.

I experienced two major CRPS symptoms: neuropathic pain and dystonia. Pain is always present in patients with CRPS, but dystonia is not. My neuropathic pain, which I defined earlier in the book as a sensation of fire ants crawling under my skin, went away completely about four months after I started with Dr. Sarno's method. It was replaced by fibromyalgia-like symptoms of widespread dull pain, which was somewhat helped by over-the-counter painkillers. The dull pain slowly faded away in another four - six months, but

I still had local pain in my hands for another few months. I used over-the-counter painkillers fairly frequently until the pain finally faded away in the fall of 2016, but I stayed away from prescription painkillers, no matter how hard it was.

The dystonia took much longer to get rid of, more than two years. It had a much longer lasting impact on me, probably because of my deeply rooted fear of becoming disabled like my Aunt Gina, but maybe because dystonia is so much harder to undo.

I consider myself 99% recovered. However, it is hard to quantify the differences between my condition today and, let's say, a year before CRPS hit me. I am pain-free, and dexterity in my hands is fully restored.

Some may say that it is unrelated to CRPS, but my sleep is much, much better than in years before CRPS. Good sleep improved the quality of my life so significantly that it could tip the scale to well over 100% recovery, if not for two very minor issues.

First, I still feel minor numbness in the tip of my left middle finger, on the inside of my middle finger, and adjacent area of the palm on my right hand. It does not bother me. It does not prevent me from doing everything I used to be able to do, and even more. Also, on occasion, I experience short-lived cramps in my hands or feet, which I didn't have before CRPS. When cramps occur, I simply try to relax, and they go away. I am in a long plateau that started about nine months ago. On several occasions I thought that I was close to getting rid of the numbness, but it has not happened yet.

As my hands started improving, my migraines and back pain that had completely disappeared during the onslaught of

CRPS now gradually returned, albeit nowhere as strong or as frequent as they used to be.

Per Dr. Sarno's observation, TMS symptoms usually present themselves one by one, replacing each other as time goes on . You get rid of one, another pops up – until you fully resolve your emotional issues. At the time of my writing this section (December 2018), I am not ready to conclude that my migraines and back pain are "replacement symptoms." I am also experiencing more outbursts of insomnia, which I can directly link to the turbulent times our country is experiencing.

Is 99% close enough to be considered 100%? My overall health is better now than it was before CRPS; however, my current symptoms signal that more meditation should be done to get rid of numbness and the last remnants of my insomnia.

Official Diagnosis

Official diagnosis from your official doctor must be taken very seriously and not ignored. Remember, Dr. Sarno never recommended his approach to patients until any potential actual structural issues were cleared. The same is done by every serious TMS professional.

Settling on the assumption that you have TMS is a very tricky and difficult step to take, and I do not want to mislead anyone. Do not seek alternative treatments if the only real solution is to turn to modern medicine. For example, if I faced a cancer diagnosis, I would not hesitate for a second to see an oncologist. However, neurological conditions could be different. They can be very debilitating but not deadly, so the risk one would take in trying the TMS route is minor compared to the risk of losing your life to cancer.

In my case, I was very lucky. My initial official diagnosis was clearly contradicting my symptoms. None of the doctors who insisted on my CTS diagnosis could explain dystonia, or hypersensitivity to cold and touch, or spreading of the symptoms to feet and ankles – these symptoms absolutely did not fit the CTS picture and motivated me to seek a more coherent conclusion.

Probably, the unresolved puzzle of my symptoms helped me resist the urge to start taking the prescription painkillers, which were so promptly offered by my doctor. Had I given in and accepted the painkillers as inevitable – my life could have turned out differently.

As a result, it was easy for me to resist the path of standard CTS treatments and defy the EMG test, which showed a significant degradation of the electrical signals in my hands. I also did some work researching a success rate of the carpal tunnel surgery and steroids and it turned out to be around 50%.

Thanks to the Google search engine, I found the Budapest Criteria, a simple diagnostic tool that clearly and unequivocally pointed to CRPS/RDS. CRPS/RDS is a rare condition, often misdiagnosed and easily overlooked by the doctors, so I am not surprised that my doctors could not figure it out. I credit the creators of the Budapest Criteria for their ability to see the forest behind the trees of the individual diagnoses. They assembled the symptoms that manifested themselves in different parts and subsystems of the body under the same roof: motor, vasomotor, sensory, edema. Each one of those would be divvied up and individually referred to various specialists - neurologist, cardiovascular specialist, rheumatologist, dermatologist - but not looked at as a multi-dimensional picture. At least this is what I observed in my experience and so did quite a few chronic pain sufferers I spoke to. The diagnosis was simple: My mindbody failed to cope with stress. However, it was not possible to be achieved by the means of our exceptionally powerful, but short-sighted healthcare system.

Interesting to note that of the many healthcare professionals who I saw for my illness, the Chinese medicine practitioners (acupressurist and acupuncturist) were the most accurate in their assessment of the cause of my symptoms, and it was a physical therapist who correctly identified the official medical diagnosis, which was later confirmed by a neurologist. Maybe you already guessed why they were closer to the truth. By the nature of their business, they must work with the entire patient; they see their patient in full, not in body parts.

Not everyone is as lucky as I was. It would be much harder for someone with severe back pain to defy an MRI exam clearly showing spine deformities, or for someone with the persistent residual pain from a real injury (a type II CRPS case) to start believing that their pain is generated by their brain for no good reason and that their structural injury has completely healed.

I have no good recommendations on this subject other than a) to look for reputable TMS practitioners and follow their advice, and b) to re-evaluate your diagnosis as you observe, learn, and understand more about yourself and your condition.

Square Peg in the Round Hole
As my friend Panda noted, I was a square peg in the round hole of the healthcare system. I really wanted to work with

the system, but the system kept pushing me back into the round hole of standard diagnoses and standard treatments. I refused to accept both the diagnosis and the treatments because they did not fit my symptoms. I heard many similar stories of patients who went from doctor to doctor, looking for a diagnosis that would take them to a successful treatment – and finding none.

As I later learned, I was lucky, because my official diagnosis had so little to do with real symptoms, because my condition was so desperate that I had no choice but fight, because I was willing to do a lot of my homework, because I had financial means to try things that were not covered by my insurance – and I succeeded by combining the tools both within and on the outside of the mainstream healthcare system.

I wonder if there are researchers out there who study the ability of our healthcare system to deliver real outcomes. I found some who evaluated efficacy of steroid injections and surgeries, but I did not find those who would cast a wider net on the overall efficacy of the most commonly used treatments.

Having been in care of various HMO (Health Management Organizations) for over 20 years, I have received dozens of follow-up surveys after my visits. They wanted to know what my wait time was, were the receptionists polite and helpful, were the facilities clean. I remember only two surveys that asked me whether I was satisfied with the care provided by the doctor. However, even those surveys were more concerned with how courteous the doctor was with me, but did not contain more important questions that I wanted to see, for example, these:

Was the health problem you complained about successfully resolved by the doctor?

Was the resolution of your complaint temporary or permanent?

Does the resolution require an ongoing treatment, such as medication, repeated surgeries, or do you feel that you no longer need supportive treatments?

Did you experience any side effects after the treatment?

Is your overall well-being better after the treatment?

I think that questions above should be asked by every patient as they seek medical help. We should be evaluating our healthcare practitioners with the expectation of return to the state of our health prior to the medical condition we sought to relieve. Our bodies and minds are designed as self-balancing systems, and we should be mostly able to recover – unless it was triggered by a major physical injury or mental trauma.

But this is not the reality we are living in. There seems to be an explosion of chronic pain in our society in the recent decades. Chronic conditions seem to appear in young people and continue to accompany us through our entire lives while we all accept inevitability of pain.

As someone who experienced those conditions since my early adulthood, I have many unanswered questions for our healthcare system:

Why is our medicine so focused on dealing with the acute conditions and ignores the ones that are deemed non-life-threatening, yet very capable of destroying one's life? How

152

often are the acute conditions the result of the chronic conditions gone too far?

Why is it acceptable that by age of 50, an average person takes several medications on an ongoing basis? Why does our society find it acceptable that so many people now must take pills to alleviate side effects of the other pills that were prescribed to them years ago?

Has anyone studied the emotional toll of a prescription drug dependency by a human being on that human being and his/her family?

Why is it easier to get a prescription for an opioid than a referral to a physical therapy? Is it due to a perceived low cost of painkillers?

Why is preventative medicine so focused on the patient's blood pressure or blood sugar but so negligent of the state of the nervous system, which may be in fact the cause of a high blood pressure or high blood sugar?

Why is it so easy to get a referral for a full bone scan and so hard to get a referral to a psychotherapist?

Considering that HMO is the most popular format for the healthcare systems in the U.S., I wonder if they are truly committed to their stated objective of providing quality healthcare at a lower cost. I wonder if, all good intentions aside, they slip into the business of providing healthcare-related services at a lower cost. But this is a question that is much bigger than the scope of my book.

Going back to my case, I came to the realization that for many years I complained about various health problems (headaches, insomnia, back pain) and accepted a position held by my doctors that my health problems were chronic and I just had to live with them and wrap my life around them. And when I found my wrist swollen and my hand extremely painful, I was ready to accept a chronic diagnosis once again. Fortunately for me, this time the pain was so bad and rapidly progressing that I refused to accept it as my new way of life. I became a square peg in the round hole. But how many of us, those square pegs are there in the system, and how many of us don't even know that they should be looking for another solution?

Confident Doctors and Over-Confident Doctors

When we are experiencing a serious health condition that is debilitating, rapidly progressing, and poorly understood, we need a doctor who we can trust. We want a doctor who is confident enough for us to believe in his/her decisions, however, not over-confident to the point of ignoring our concerns and swatting away our questions. We need a doctor who would be willing to accept us as intelligent and equal partners in making decisions for our health. And, of course, we need a doctor who has a gift of compassion.

A non-confident doctor would be playing a medical ping-pong of a sort, sending you around to the specialists in hopes that they would make a diagnosis, and would do so endlessly and without a clear plan. It also could be that a non-confident doctor would be hiding behind the mask of over-confidence, presenting him/herself as such out of fear of being challenged by the patient.

I also quickly discovered that, once misdiagnosed by an over-confident doctor, it is very difficult to remove that diagnosis from your file and it may affect the treatments and procedures that you are prescribed. No matter how many times my symptoms and later my recovery disproved the carpal tunnel syndrome diagnosis, it is still on my chart. Beware that time is of the essence and be ready at some point to confront your doctor if you feel that a vital decision must be made. At that point, be ready to look for another physician if you feel that you have gotten nowhere.

In my case, I quickly realized that while my primary physician Dr. B was just fine when I was healthy and saw her for a physical exam once a year, at the time of a crisis she was unhelpful. It is very difficult to change doctors when you are very ill, but as hard as it is, change may lead to a positive outcome and is worth trying.

My advice is: Don't wait for the crisis, find a good doctor before you get sick!

Faith, Patience, Courage

Finally, these are the key points. To succeed in beating down your TMS, you need to be patient and have faith in yourself.

Most importantly, you need to believe that rather than coping with chronic pain, you should be aiming to get rid of it. There is a fundamental difference between pain management and healing from pain. Pain management, as taught in pain management clinics, teaches you to live with pain, to settle, to accept your incapacitation. Focus on healing from pain takes you to the goal of living without pain, of not settling, on getting your life back.

But even more so, you need to look inside yourself, to have courage to view and understand your personality traits as an outsider, without personal attachment or resentment. It comes with self-awareness and mindfulness.

The more you practice mindfulness and observe your own behavior, the sooner your meditation practice will be able to deal with what is on your mind. As you meditate, you would recognize the thoughts flashing through your brain, pick them apart - and understand them. Often just a basic awareness is enough for your brain to stop sending the signals of pain into your body. A perfect example of this awareness are Dr. Sarno's lectures, books, and CDs, which set his patients on the path of their mindfulness journey. Many people healed using his method by just reading his book – isn't that a remarkable proof of the power of mind?

And the last point is for the skeptics who still doubt the TMS concept. Let's assume all these TMS successes are purely a placebo effect. In that case, the healing power of placebo can only be explained by the act of God or by the act of a patient's mind. Regardless of whether it is me controlling my mind or God's hand - you decide - the outcome is a successful recovery of the patient.

If I were to choose between a surgery with a success rate of 50% or a placebo with a similar success rate, I would go for a placebo in a heartbeat. It costs me less, it does not have side effects, and it gives me a sense of personal growth. On the downside, it drives less business the way of the surgeons – but is it a bad thing?

So, if you or your loved one decided to give the TMS approach a try upon reading my book – I consider my time and effort well spent. The mindfulness journey never ends, as we never stop to grow as human beings.

Safe travels and best of luck, my reader!

Glossary

CRPS (Complex Regional Pain Syndrome), previously known as RSD (Reflex Sympathetic Dystrophy), is considered a rare disease (200,000 cases in the U.S.). It is associated with severe, chronic pain; various pathologies affecting the nervous system, soft tissues and musculoskeletal system; and, in some cases extreme swelling and bone, skin, and bodily deformities. The pain experienced by CRPS patients is so extreme that it is measured on its own scale, where childbirth is rated at 40 points and CRPS pain at 50. Childbirth lasts for hours, while CRPS pain is chronic and may persist for decades. Untreated, CRPS progresses from stage 1 to stage 4, when even amputations of the limbs are recommended, in hopes of stopping the pain – often unsuccessfully. Treatments available for CRPS range from opioids to nerve blockages, but those are mostly supportive therapies that generally do not result in a full remission. It is not unusual for symptoms to return after a short break. Loss of employment, income, medical insurance, and social status are frequent outcomes for CRPS patients and can be devastating to the patients and their families.

CTS - Carpal Tunnel Syndrome. Defined by the National Institute of Health as a condition that occurs when "the median nerve, which runs from the forearm into the palm of the hand, becomes pressed or squeezed at the wrist." Carpal tunnel is "a narrow, rigid passageway of ligament and bones at the base of the hand—houses the median nerve and the tendons that bend the fingers."

Extinction Burst. Extinction burst is defined by Dr. Sarno as a sudden increase in pain symptoms in the chronic pain patients during their recovery from chronic pain. While the nature of those bursts of pain is not well understood, the experience seems to be very common among those who follow the TMS approach.

EMG – Electromyography. Diagnostic procedure that evaluates health of muscles.

Budapest Criteria. Also known as Budapest Protocol. Set of criteria allowing to make a clinical diagnosis of CRPS. Adopted by the authoritative group of pain medicine specialists to establish simple, consistent, and expedient method of diagnosing CRPS.

Budapest Protocol. See Budapest Criteria.

RSD (Reflex Sympathetic Dystrophy) – see CRPS

TMS - Tension Myositis Syndrome. Term initially coined by Dr. Sarno to define emotionally induced pain. It is now often referred to as **The Mindbody Syndrome**, which more accurately reflects the underlying nature of TMS.

Bibliography

[1] B. E. a. P. B. Dexter Louie, "Long-term outcomes of carpal tunnel release: a critical review of the literature," 22 June 2012. [Online]. Available: https://www.ncbi.nlm.nih.gov/pmc/articles/PMC3418353/.

[2] "Carpal Tunnel Syndrome Fact Sheet," 13 August 2019. [Online]. Available: https://www.ninds.nih.gov/Disorders/Patient-Caregiver-Education/Fact-Sheets/Carpal-Tunnel-Syndrome-Fact-Sheet. [Accessed 2019].

[3] "Carpal tunnel syndrome: How effective are corticosteroid treatments?," 16 November 2017. [Online]. Available: https://www.ncbi.nlm.nih.gov/books/NBK279598/.

[4] "Cure Dystonia Now," [Online]. Available: www.curedystonianow.org.

[5] "National Health Service of UK," [Online]. Available: https://www.nhs.uk/conditions/complex-regional-pain-syndrome/treatment/.

[6] M. a. H. J. M. P. Leslie J Cloud, "Treatment Strategies For Dystonia," [Online]. Available: https://www.ncbi.nlm.nih.gov/pmc/articles/PMC3495548/.

[7] M. Gaurav Gupta, "Complex Regional Pain Syndromes," 2018. [Online]. Available: https://emedicine.medscape.com/article/1145318-overview.

[8] ,. F. B. J. S. a. U. H. Maria M. Wertli, "Usefulness of bone scintigraphy for the diagnosis of Complex Regional Pain Syndrome 1: A systematic review and Bayesian meta-analysis," 16 March 2017. [Online]. Available: https://www.ncbi.nlm.nih.gov/pmc/articles/PMC5354289/.

[9] J. E. Sarno, Mindbody Prescription, Warner Books, Inc., 1999.

[10] R. Sapolsky, Why Zebras Don't Get Ulcers, 2004.

[11] "What Jobs Cause Carpal Tunnel Syndrome?," [Online]. Available: http://www.workers-comp-news.com/jobs-carpal-tunnel.php.

[12] P. C. a. T. R. Renee J. Hill, "Rethinking the Psychogenic Model of Complex Regional Pain Syndrome: Somatoform Disorders and Complex Regional Pain Syndrome," 2012. [Online]. Available: https://www.ncbi.nlm.nih.gov/pmc/articles/PMC3821113/.

[13] "Complex Regional Pain Syndrome Fact Sheet," [Online]. Available: https://www.ninds.nih.gov/Disorders/Patient-Caregiver-Education/Fact-

Sheets/Complex-Regional-Pain-Syndrome-Fact-Sheet. [Accessed 2019].

[14] "Meditation: In Depth," 2 April 2016. [Online]. Available: https://nccih.nih.gov/health/meditation/overview.htm.

[15] S. Ozanich., The Great Pain Deception, 2011.

[16] C. Weekes, "Hope And Help For Your Nerves. Audio CD," 2012.

[17] P. Joaquin Farias, "Limitless. How Your Movements Can Heal Your Brain," 2016. [Online]. Available: https://www.fariastechnique.com/focal-dystonia-ebooks/limitless-how-your-movements-can-change-your-brain-an-essay-on-the-neurodynamics-of-dystonia.

[18] T. J. Kaptchuk, The Web That Has No Weaver : Understanding Chinese Medicine., McGraw-Hill Education, 2002.